Nutrition and Fitness: Evolutionary Aspects, Children's Health, Programs and Policies

World Review of Nutrition and Dietetics

Vol. 81

Series Editor

Artemis P. Simopoulos
The Center for Genetics, Nutrition and Health,
Washington, D.C., USA

Advisory Board

Åke Bruce, Sweden
Ji Di Chen, China
Jean-Claude Dillon, France
J.E. Dutra de Oliveira, Brazil
Claudio Galli, Italy
Ghafoorunissa, India
Demetre Labadarios, South Africa
Eleazar Lara-Pantin, Venezuela
Paul J. Nestel, Australia
Konstantin Pavlou, Greece
A. Rérat, France
V. Rogozkin, Russia
Michihiro Sugano, Japan
Naomi Trostler, Israel
Ricardo Uauy-Dagach, Chile

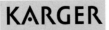

Basel · Freiburg · Paris · London · New York ·
New Delhi · Bangkok · Singapore · Tokyo · Sydney

3rd International Conference on Nutrition and Fitness,
Athens, May 24–27, 1996

....

Nutrition and Fitness: Evolutionary Aspects, Children's Health, Programs and Policies

Volume Editor   *A.P. Simopoulos*
The Center for Genetics, Nutrition and Health,
Washington, D.C.

7 figures, and 31 tables, 1997

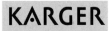

Basel · Freiburg · Paris · London · New York ·
New Delhi · Bangkok · Singapore · Tokyo · Sydney

••••••••••••••••••••••••

Additional proceedings from the conference are published in volume 82 of this series.

Library of Congress Cataloging-in-Publication Data
International Conference on Nutrition and Fitness (3rd: 1996: Athens, Greece)
Nutrition and fitness: evolutionary aspects, children's health, programs, and
policies: 3rd International Conference on Nutrition and Fitness, Athens, May 24–27, 1996 /
[editor, Artemis P. Simopoulos].
(World review of nutrition and dietetics; vol. 81)
Includes bibliographical references and index.
1. Nutrition – Congresses. 2. Nutrition policy – Congresses. 3. Children – Nutrition – Congresses.
I. Simopoulos, Artemis P., 1933–. II. Series.
QP141.A1W59 vol. 81
612.3 s–dc21
[613.2]
ISBN 3–8055–6452–X (hardcover; alk. paper)

Bibliographic Indices. This publication is listed in bibliographic services, including Current Contents® and Index Medicus.

Drug Dosage. The authors and the publisher have exerted every effort to ensure that drug selection and dosage set forth in this text are in accord with current recommendations and practice at the time of publication. However, in view of ongoing research, changes in government regulations, and the constant flow of information relating to drug therapy and drug reactions, the reader is urged to check the package insert for each drug for any change in indications and dosage and for added warnings and precautions. This is particularly important when the recommended agent is a new and/or infrequently employed drug.

© Copyright 1997 by S. Karger AG, P.O. Box, CH–4009 Basel (Switzerland)
Printed in Switzerland on acid-free paper by Reinhardt Druck, Basel.
ISBN 3–8055–6452–X

••••••••••••••••••••••••••

The proceedings of the conference are dedicated
to the concept of positive health as enunciated by the
Hippocratic physicians (5th century BC).

Positive health requires a knowledge of man's primary constitution
(which today we call genetics) and of the powers of various foods,
both those natural to them and those resulting from human skill
(today's processed food).
But eating alone is not enough for health.
There must also be exercise,
of which the effects must likewise be known.
The combination of these two things makes regimen,
when proper attention is given to the season of the year,
the changes of the winds,
the age of the individual and the situation of his home.
If there is any deficiency in food or exercise the body will fall sick.

Contents

IX   **Conference Organization**

XI   **Preface**

1   **Declaration of Olympia on Nutrition and Fitness**
Ancient Olympia, Greece, May 28–29, 1996

10   **Declaration of Olympia on Nutrition and Fitness**
Ancient Olympia, Greece, May 26, 1992

12   **Conference Resolutions**
Ancient Olympia, Greece, May 26, 1988

13   **Diet, Physical Activity, and Health: Policies for the New Millennium**
Keynote Address
Lee, P.R.; Meyers, L.D. (Washington, D.C.)

Part 1: Genetics, Nutrition, Physical Activity and Health

24   **Summary of Part I**
Simopoulos, A.P. (Washington, D.C.); Eaton, S.B. (Atlanta, Ga.)

26   **Evolutionary Aspects of Diet: Old Genes, New Fuels**
Nutritional Changes Since Agriculture
Eaton, S.B. (Atlanta, Ga.); Cordain, L. (Fort Collins, Colo.)

38   **Paleonutrition and Modern Nutrition**
Phillipson, C. (Athens)

49   **Evolutionary Aspects of Exercise**
Cordain, L.; Gotshall, R.W. (Fort Collins, Colo.); Eaton, S.B. (Atlanta, Ga.)

61   **Genetic Variation: Nutrients, Physical Activity and Gene Expression**
Simopoulos, A.P. (Washington, D.C.)

72   **Genetics, Response to Exercise, and Risk Factors:
The HERITAGE Family Study**
Wilmore, J.H. (Austin, Tex.); Leon, A.S. (Minneapolis, Minn.);
Rao, D.C. (St. Louis, Mo.); Skinner, J.S. (Bloomington, Ind.); Gagnon, J.;
Bouchard, C. (Québec)

Part 2: Exercise and Children's Health

84 **Summary of Part 2**
Grave, G.D. (Bethesda, Md.)

90 **Nutritional Needs of the Exercising Child**
Stallings, V.A. (Philadelphia, Pa.)

98 **Health-Related Physical Activity and Fitness among European Children and Adolescents**
Oja, P. (Tampere)

Part 3: National Programs and Policies Promoting Better Nutrition, Physical Fitness and Sports for All

105 **Summary of Part 3**
Bourne, P.G. (Washington, D.C.)

108 **Nutrition and Physical Activity Perspectives for All Americans: Government and Private Sector Partnerships for the Twenty-First Century**
Lee, P.R.; Meyers, L.D. (Washington, D.C.)

114 **National Policies Promoting Better Nutrition, Physical Fitness and Sports for All in China**
Chen, J.D. (Beijing)

122 **National Programs and Policies Promoting Better Nutrition, Physical Fitness and Sports for All: Experiences from Africa**
Siandwazi, C. (Arusha)

128 **National Programs and Policies Promoting Better Nutrition, Fitness and Sports for All in Greece**
Matalas, A.-L. (Athens)

136 **National Policies for Promoting Physical Activity, Physical Fitness and Better Nutrition in Europe**
van Mechelen, W. (Amsterdam)

148 **National Policies Promoting Better Nutrition, Physical Fitness and Sports for All in Australia**
Truswell, A.S. (Sydney)

160 **Is Physical Activity Promotion on the Primary Health Care Agenda?**
Gould, M.M.; Iliffe, S.; Thorogood, M. (London)

167 **Author Index**

168 **Subject Index**

....
Conference Organization

Conference Cochairs
Artemis P. Simopoulos, MD (USA)
Konstantinos N. Pavlou, ScD (Greece)

Executive Committee

Artemis P. Simopoulos, MD (USA), Chairman

Konstantinos N. Pavlou, ScD (Greece), Cochairman

Peter Bourne, MD (USA)

Regina Casper, MD, PhD (USA)

Ji Di Chen, MD (China)

Nicholas T. Christakos, Esq. (USA)

J.E. Dutra-de-Oliveira, MD (Brazil)

Sotiris Kitrilakis (Greece)

Eleazar Lara-Pantin, MD (Venezuela)

Alexander Leaf, MD (USA)

Argiris Mitsou, MD (Greece)

Aulikki Nissinen, MD, PhD (Finland)

Fernandos Serpieris (Greece)

Kihumbu Thairu, PhD (Kenya)

A. Stewart Truswell, PhD (Australia)

Ricardo Uauy, MD, PhD (Chile)

Clyde Williams, PhD (UK)

Organized by
The Center for Genetics, Nutrition and Health
The Hellenic Sports Research Institute
The Olympic Athletic Center of Athens, Spyros Louis
College of Sport Sciences

Under the Patronage of
The General Secretariat of Athletics of Greece – Ministry of Culture
Food and Agriculture Organization of the United Nations
World Health Organization
International Olympic Academy
Hellenic Ministry of Health

Preface

The international conferences on Nutrition and Fitness are held in Greece the last week in May every 4 years prior to the Olympic games. The Third International Conference on Nutrition and Fitness was held May 24–27, 1996 in Athens, Greece. Following the conference in Athens, members of the Executive Committee, Session Chairmen, and some of the sponsors met at the International Olympic Academy at Ancient Olympia, May 28–29, to develop the 1996 'Declaration of Olympia on Nutrition and Fitness'. The third international conference, as the two previous ones, is dedicated to the concept of Positive Health as enunciated by Hippocrates in 480 BC:

'Positive health requires a knowledge of man's primary constitution (which today we call genetics) and of the powers of various foods, both those natural to them and those resulting from human skill (today's processed food). But eating alone is not enough for health. There must also be exercise, of which the effects must likewise be known. The combination of these two things makes regimen, when proper attention is given to the season of the year, the changes of the winds, the age of the individual and the situation of his home. If there is any deficiency in food or exercise the body will fall sick.'

It is indeed amazing how modern and timely the concept of Positive Health sounds today. Using the techniques of molecular biology in genetic studies, it is clear that both nutrients and physical activity influence gene expression. At the same time, clinical studies indicate that the response to diet depends on our genetic profile. Genetic variation or polymorphisms contribute to human diversity and human's response to diet. Furthermore, gene frequencies differ in various populations as shown by the frequency of apolipoprotein (Apo) E4 associated with hypercholesterolemia and coronary heart disease (New Guinea, 37%; Nigeria, 30%; Caucasians, 15% (average); Finland, 22.7%; Sweden, 20%; Italy, 9.4%) and the vitamin D receptor (VDR) allele related to osteoporosis (designated BB genotype) (Cambridge, UK, 15.4%; China 0.0%; The Gambia, 3.3%; African-Americans, Boston, USA, 8.3%), just to name two well-studied genetic polymorphisms. Therefore, universal dietary recommendations are not appropriate for the prevention of chronic diseases; neither should data relating diet to chronic diseases be extrapolated from one population to another.

The objectives of the conference were to:

Review and critique the latest scientific information on nutrition and fitness, taking into consideration genetic endowment, adaptation throughout the life cycle and the nutritional factors that contribute to fitness, specifically, the effect of the various dietary sources of energy on energy expenditure, exercise and performance.

Determine the relationship of nutrition and fitness to chronic diseases, particularly, the metabolic changes that occur with the type and amount of physical activity for the prevention and management of cardiovascular disease, obesity, diabetes, osteoporosis, and cancer.

Consider the psychosocial and other determinants of physical activity throughout the life cycle including intervention strategies, and emphasize healthy lifestyles consistent with proper nutrition and fitness.

Stimulate national governments and the private sector to coordinate and thus maximize their efforts to develop programs that encourage proper nutrition and participation in sports activities by all, throughout the life cycle, to achieve their potential in fitness and thus increase the pool of young athletes, from whom the elite athlete will be forthcoming.

The objectives of the conference were indeed fulfilled, as shown by the excellent papers included in the two volumes of the proceedings. Four hundred and eighty participants attended the conference from 31 countries representing all continents. The scientific program consisted of 30 invited papers, 21 oral presentations, and 50 poster abstracts.

The proceedings of the conference consist of two volumes in this series, volumes 81 and 82, which include the invited papers and selected oral presentations. Volume 81 is entitled 'Nutrition and Fitness: Evolutionary Aspects, Children's Health, Programs and Policies' and volume 82 is entitled 'Nutrition and Fitness: Metabolic and Behavioral Aspects in Health and Disease'. Volume 81 consists of three parts. Part 1: Genetics, Nutrition, Physical Activity and Health; Part 2: Exercise and Children's Health; and Part 3: National Programs and Policies Promoting Better Nutrition, Physical Fitness and Sports for All. Volume 82 consists also of three parts: Part 1: Nutrition and Physical Activity; Part 2: Exercise Psychology Throughout the Life Cycle; and Part 3: Exercise Prescription. Each part is preceded by a summary of the session. The 'Declaration of Olympia on Nutrition and Fitness' (1996) appears in both volumes immediately after the preface. For the sake of continuity, the points of the declaration from the second (1992), and the resolutions of the first conference on nutrition and fitness (1988), follow. The keynote address given by Dr. Philip

Lee, Assistant Secretary for Health, US Department of Health and Human Services appears next, followed by the session summaries and papers.

Part 1 of volume 81 consists of the papers on evolutionary aspects of diet, evolutionary aspects of exercise, genetics, nutrition, physical activity and health, and the 'Heritage' study which investigates the genetic basis for differences in response to exercise and the modification by exercise of genetic risks for coronary artery disease. Anatomically, modern human beings first appeared in the fossil record 90,000–100,000 years ago in the Near East and Africa, and the first truly modern humans, complete with art, culture and sophisticated tools are recognizable by 40,000 years ago. Until 10,000 years ago, all hominids were hunters-gatherers. Consequently, by studying the physical activity patterns to which we are genetically adapted, insight can be gained in determining optimal exercise levels for modern sedentary societies.

For the hunter-gatherer, energy expenditure was directly linked to food procurement. Similar to all other organisms, the human genome was shaped by environmental selective pressures over eons of evolutionary experience. Technological achievement and social organization have disrupted the evolutionary relationship between food procurement and energy expenditure. Contemporary man's biology has become so disordered that physiological and biochemical risk factors affecting the cardiovascular system, the skeleton, and carbohydrate metabolism, are now very common for the first time. In the development of chronic diseases, departure from dietary and exercise patterns that prevailed during evolution plays a fundamental role. Mitochondrial DNA evidence suggests that the modern human genome is almost identical to that of paleolithic humans who lived 40,000 years ago. Therefore, the exercise capacities and requirements of modern humans remain similar to those which had been originally selected by evolution for stone age humans living in a hunting and gathering environment.

In order to understand why a causal relationship exists among exercise, nutrition, health and fitness, they must be examined from an evolutionary perspective. Because similar beneficial metabolic changes occur through dietary manipulation or physical activity, the effects of exercise on children's health are presented in part 2.

The volume concludes with national programs and policies promoting better nutrition, physical fitness and sports for all. Although the papers included in part 3 represent the US, Europe, England, Greece, Africa, Australia/ New Zealand, and China, there were a number of posters on this topic from many countries. It was agreed that each county needs to combine their nutrition and physical activity programs both for the prevention and management of diseases. There has been a decrease in physical activity programs that mandate physical activities in primary and secondary schools in all countries represented at the conference. However, efforts are being made to both increase and coordinate government programs with programs provided by both non-profit and for-profit organizations. There were papers that evaluated health programs promoting physical activity within medical clinics. The evaluation shows that in England concern was expressed about 'medicalization of lifestyles'. Obviously, different models will have to be developed that are appropriate for each country or region. Greece, more than any other country, has mandatory physical activities three times per week at both primary and secondary schools, but it will have to develop a model that includes diet along with exercise.

Volume 81 should be of interest to geneticists, anthropologists, exercise physiologists, nutritionists, dietitians, psychologists, psychiatrists, pediatricians, internists, general practitioners, health care providers, industrial scientists, policy makers, and national and international governmental organizations.

Artemis P. Simopoulos, MD

Simopoulos AP (ed): Nutrition and Fitness: Evolutionary Aspects, Children's Health, Programs and Policies. World Rev Nutr Diet. Basel, Karger, 1997, vol 81, pp 1–9

······················

Declaration of Olympia on Nutrition and Fitness

Ancient Olympia, Greece, May 28–29, 1996

Background

The International Conferences on Nutrition and Fitness are held in Greece every 4 years in the spring prior to the Olympic Games. Following each conference, a declaration is developed at a special meeting at the International Olympic Academy to update advice on nutrition and fitness for all. The proceedings of the conferences are published in the scientific literature listed on page 9.

The Third International Conference on Nutrition and Fitness was held at the Olympic Athletic Center of Athens 'Spyros Louis', May 24–27, 1996, in Athens, Greece. Four hundred and eighty participants from 31 countries attended the conference. Following the conference, an international panel composed of members of the conference Executive Committee, along with the session chairs, met at the International Olympic Academy at Ancient Olympia to develop the 'Declaration of Olympia on Nutrition and Fitness' for 1996.

This international panel agreed that on the occasion of the 100th anniversary of the Olympic Games, it is important to reaffirm the concepts of positive health postulated by Hippocrates and to reassess their relevance to the Olympic ideal and the health of the world's population. The concept of Positive Health, as enunciated by Hippocrates, is based on the interaction of genetics, diet and physical activity.

'Positive health requires a knowledge of man's primary constitution (which today we call genetics) and of the powers of various foods, both those natural to them and those resulting from human skill (today's processed food). But eating alone is not enough for health. There must also be exercise, of which the effects must likewise be known. The combination of these two things makes regimen, when proper attention is given to the season

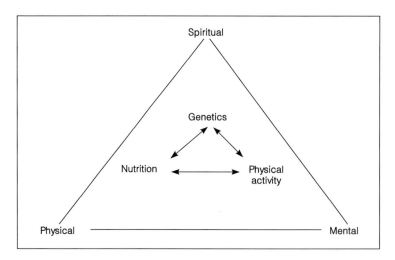

Fig. 1. The interaction of genetics, nutrition and physical activity influences the spiritual, mental and physical aspects of health.

of the year, the changes of the winds, the age of the individual and the situation of his home. If there is any deficiency in food or exercise the body will fall sick.' (480 BC)

Among the Greeks, the concept of positive health was important and occupied much of their thinking. Those who had the means and the leisure applied themselves to maintaining positive health, which they often conceived esthetically, and to this end put themselves into the hands of trainers who subjected them to a regimen. Training for war and athletic competition was of course well known among them. Health was an excellence in its own right, the physical counterpart and condition of mental activation. The details of the regimen practiced for health were an important part of Greek medicine. The Concept of Positive Health may be represented by a triangle involving genetics, nutrition and physical activity that influence the spiritual, mental and physical aspects of health (fig. 1).

Genetic Variation, Nutrition, Physical Activity, and Health

The interaction between genetic and environmental factors influences human development and is the foundation for health and disease. Genetic factors define susceptibility to disease and environmental factors determine which genetically susceptible individuals will be affected. Nutrition and physical activity (exercise) are two of the most important environmental factors in maintaining health and well being.

Each human being, in being unique, is exceptional in some way. Individuality is determined by genes, constitutional factors (age, sex, developmental stage, parental factors), and environmental factors (diet, physical activity, socioeconomic status, occupation, education, time, geography, and climate). Genetic variation is due to variants at a single locus, or polymorphisms, that form the basis of human diversity, including the ability to handle environmental challenges. How extensively variable the human species is depends on the methods used for the determination of variability. At the DNA level, there is a great deal of variation, whereas at the level of protein diversity, there is much less. In all animals, including humans and practically all other organisms examined, 30% of loci have polymorphic variants in the population. An average individual is heterozygous at about 10% of the loci. Alleles that confer selective advantage in the heterozygous state are likely to have increased in prevalence because of positive selection acting on variants. Changes in the nutritional environment and the type and degree of physical activity affect heritability of the variant phenotypes that are dependent, to a lesser or greater degree, on these environmental variables for their expression.

Genetic variation influences the response to diet. Nutrients and physical activity influence gene expression. In many conditions, proper diet and exercise have similar beneficial effects, and their effects may be additive. Because of differences in gene frequency, dietary habits, and activity levels, universal dietary and physical activity recommendations are not appropriate. Instead, knowledge of specific genes and response to exercise and diet should guide advice for health in the prevention and management of chronic diseases.

Diet

The purpose of diet is to supply energy and nutrients required for optimal health. Energy intake must be balanced against physical activity. Over 800 million humans are chronically energy deficient, but obesity is rampant in many industrialized societies.

Macronutrients

Fat is a concentrated energy source, but in affluent populations, excess fat promotes chronic degenerative diseases. In such circumstances, total fat intake should be reduced, mainly by decreases in saturated and trans fatty acids. In energy-deficient populations, an increased fat intake may be necessary to enhance energy availability and to insure absorption of fat soluble vitamins, but such increases should avoid adding saturated fats where practicable. All populations need essential polyunsaturated fatty acids for mental and cardiovascular health. An omega-6:omega-3 fatty acid ratio of 5:1 or less appears desirable.

Carbohydrate containing foods and soluble and insoluble fiber are needed for energy intake and normal bodily function.

Protein intake should be adequate for normal growth and development and in adults for maintenance of body structures.

Micronutrients

Adequate balanced micronutrient intake should be provided commensurate with emerging understanding of their need. Since the most extensive nutritional influences throughout the world are related to inadequacies of micronutrients, special attention should be directed to correcting these deficiencies: 2 thousand million persons are anemic and 1 thousand million are at risk of iodine deficiency. 40 million children suffer vitamin A deficiency. Understanding of micronutrient functions is currently increasing, and health workers should keep up-to-date with this new knowledge regarding both deficiencies and optimal requirements, e.g. the need for unitary ratios of calcium and magnesium in the diet. The variety of foods in the diets helps to maintain adequate micronutrient intake. Most populations would benefit from an increased intake of fruits and vegetables.

Physical Activity

A wealth of scientific reports points to the inescapable conclusion that human fitness and health improve when sedentary individuals begin to exercise. Although low physical activity levels most frequently occur in more industrialized, affluent nations, this behavior is becoming increasingly common in developing countries as well. Because mechanization and industrialization have reduced occupational physical activity levels, a need exists to supplement with additional daily physical activities designed to improve health and fitness.

A wide variety of fitness parameters, including aerobic capacity, muscular strength and endurance, coordination, flexibility and body composition improve with increases in activity levels. Perhaps more importantly, indices of human health also improve. Three of the most common chronic degenerative diseases of westernized nations (hypertension, coronary heart disease, and non-insulin-dependent diabetes mellitus) are increasingly being recognized as diseases of insulin resistance. In all three cases, physical activity clearly has been shown to reduce the severity, and outcome of these diseases. Physical activity also has a well-known role in preventing and reducing obesity and also

Table 1. Defining physical activity

1	Nonlabor daily physical activities
	Feeding
	Bodily functions (e.g. temperature regulation, heart rate, breathing rate)
	All daily nonlabor minimum physical activities necessary for life maintenance
2	Labor physical activities
	Industrial
	Agriculture
	Carpentry
	Homecare, etc.
3	Leisure-recreational (exercise), low-to-moderate intensity of physical activities
	Walking
	Dancing
	Hiking
	Bowling
	Cycling
	Golf, etc.

exerts a beneficial influence upon insulin metabolism. Furthermore, increased levels of physical activity positively impact virtually all chronic diseases, including, but not limited to stroke, peripheral artery disease, coronary heart disease, chronic obstructive pulmonary disease, osteoporosis, and some forms of cancer. For previously sedentary individuals, even nontaxing physical activities such as walking, gardening, bicycling, and swimming can elicit improved health, and reduce all causes of morbidity and mortality. Table 1 lists the types of physical activity. Sports training physical activities should include daily training programs in preparation for competition. Health-promoting physical activities aim at promoting growth, improving body functions and protecting from illness. Exercise prescription (regimen) as a means of treating or reversing various diseases should be considered as an essential therapeutic component.

Education

Education about nutrition and physical activity needs to be adapted to each country and to different populations and cultures. Education about the beneficial physical and psychological effects of proper nutrition and physical activity in health and disease needs to be directed at all age groups – children, adults, and the elderly – since research has shown that awareness of the benefits of physical activity is correlated with actual physical activity. Education needs to address the detrimental effects of sedentary life-styles, undernutrition and malnutrition, in particular for children. Education about opportunities to obtain proper nutrition and to carry out physical activity is important in view of findings that actual increases in elective physical activity depend on accessibility.

Education should reach people through various channels – the mass media, print, television, and radio – at worksites, and in the community in order to reach everybody in the population. Another means to achieve education would be through role models in the family, schools, sports, and entertainment. Institutions such as schools can set examples for proper nutrition and physical activity. The food and sports foods industry needs to be cognizant of the scientific evidence regarding optimal nutrition and physical activity levels. Another means of education would be the labelling of the nutritional composition of all foods sold.

There is a particular need for education of health professionals and health workers, nutrition and sport scientists, and educators.

Declaration

(1) Nutrition and physical activity interact in harmony and are the two most important positive factors that contribute to metabolic fitness and health interacting with the genetic endowment of the individual. Genes define opportunities for health and susceptibility to disease, while environmental factors determine which susceptible individuals will develop illness. Therefore, individual variation may need to be considered to achieve optimal health and to correct disorders associated with micronutrient deficiency, dietary imbalance and a sedentary lifestyle.

(2) Every child and adult needs sufficient food and physical activity to express their genetic potential for growth, development, and health. Insufficient consumption of energy, protein, essential fatty acids, vitamins (particularly vitamins A, C, D, E and the B complex) and minerals (particularly calcium, iron, iodine, potassium and zinc), and inadequate opportunities for physical activity impair the attainment of overall health and musculoskeletal function.

(3) Balancing physical activity and good nutrition for fitness is best illustrated by the concept of energy intake and output. For sedentary populations, physical activity must be increased; for populations engaging in intense occupational and/or recreational physical activities, food consumption may need to be increased to meet their energy needs.

(4) Nutrient intakes should match more closely human evolutionary heritage. The choice of foods should lead to a diverse diet high in fruits and vegetables and rich in essential nutrients, particularly protective antioxidants and essential fatty acids.

(5) The current level of physical activity should match more closely our genetic endowment. Reestablishment of regular physical activity into everyday life on a daily basis is essential for physical, mental and spiritual well-being. For all ages and both genders the physical activity should be appropriately vigorous and of sufficient duration, frequency, and intensity, using large muscle groups rhythmically and repetitively. Special attention to adequate nutrition should be given to competitive athletes.

(6) The attainment of metabolic fitness through energy balance, good nutrition and physical activity, reduces the risk of and forms the treatment framework for many modern lifestyle diseases such as diabetes mellitus, hypertension, osteoporosis, some cancers, obesity, and cardiovascular disorders. Metabolic fitness maintains and improves musculoskeletal function, mobility, and the activities of daily living into old age.

(7) Education regarding healthy nutrition and physical activity must begin early and continue throughout life. Nutrition and physical activity must be interwoven into the curriculum of school age children and of educators, nutritionists and other health professionals. Positive role models must be developed and promoted by society and the media.

(8) Major personal behavioral changes supported by the family, the community, and societal resources are necessary to reject unhealthy lifestyles and to embrace an active lifestyle and good nutrition.

(9) National governments and the private sector must coordinate their efforts to encourage good nutrition and physical activity throughout the life cycle and thus increase the pool of physically fit individuals who emulate the Olympic ideal.

(10) The ancient Greeks (Hellenes) attained a high level of civilization based on good nutrition, regular physical activity, and intellectual development. They strove for excellence in mind and body. Modern men, women, and children can emulate this Olympic ideal and become swifter, stronger and fitter through regular physical activity and good nutrition.

Distribution of the Declaration

The declaration has been published worldwide in newsletters, magazines and journals. It has been translated into the Olympic languages of Chinese, French, Greek, Russian and Spanish. The ten points of the declaration have been printed in these languages. The Executive Committee wishes to encourage the translation and distribution of the declaration worldwide. The copyright is held by the Executive Committee of the Conference.

The declaration was developed at Ancient Olympia, May 28–29, 1996 by the following persons:

Alexander Leaf, MD(Cochairman), USA

Peter G. Bourne, MD (Cochairman), USA, UK

Richard B. Birrer, MD (Secretary), USA

Regina Casper, MD, PhD, USA

Ji Di Chen, MD, China

William Clay, FAO, United Nations

Loren Cordain, PhD, USA

S. Boyd Eaton, MD, USA

Gilman Grave, MD, USA

Philip R. Lee, MD, USA

Konstantinos N. Pavlou, ScD, Greece

Catherine Siandwazi, Tanzania, UK

Artemis P. Simopoulos, MD, USA

The Fourth International Conference on Nutrition and Fitness will be held in Greece in the Spring of the year 2000, and subsequent conferences every 4 years in Greece.

Acknowledgement

The Third International Conference on Nutrition and Fitness was organized by The Center for Genetics, Nutrition and Health (USA); The Hellenic Sports Research Institute; and the College of Sports Science (Greece). The conference was under the patronage of The General Secretariat of Athletics of Greece – Ministry of Culture; Food and Agriculture Organization of the United Nations–FAO; World Health Organization–WHO; International Olympic Academy–IOA, and the Hellenic Ministry of Health. The conference was cosponsored by Harokopio University (Greece), The Center for Genetics, Nutrition and Health (USA); The Ministry of Health and Social Services (Greece), General Secretariat of Athletics of Greece; The Hellenic Sports Research Institute; The Olympic Athletic Center of Athens, Spyros Louis; The President's Council on Physical Fitness and Sports (USA); National Institute of Child Health and Human Development–NIH (USA); American Association for World Health–AAWH; International Union of Nutritional Sciences-IUNS; The American Institute for Cancer Research; Amway Corporation; Campbell Soup Company; Mars, Inc.; Mitchell Energy & Development Corporation (USA); National Dairy Council (USA); Nestec Ltd, Nestle Research Center; Nutrilite, Inc.; Egnatia Epirus Foundation; Macedonian Wine Route, A-B Vasilopoulos; and Peloponnese – Mediterranean Specialities. The Executive Committee would like to thank the above patrons and sponsors for their ongoing support of the conferences.

Literature

1 Simopoulos AP (ed): Proceedings of the First International Conference on Nutrition and Fitness. Am J Clin Nutr 1989;49(suppl):909–1124.
2 Simopoulos AP, Pavlou KN (eds): Volume I. Nutrition and Fitness for Athletes. Proceedings of the Second International Conference on Nutrition and Fitness. World Rev Nutr Diet. Basel, Karger, 1993, vol 71.
3 Simopoulos AP (ed): Volume II. Nutrition and Fitness in Health and Disease. Proceedings of the Second International Conference on Nutrition and Fitness. World Rev Nutr Diet. Basel, Karger, 1993, vol 72.
4 Simopoulos AP (ed): Volume I. Nutrition and Fitness: Evolutionary Aspects, Children, Health, Policies and Programs. Proceedings of the Third International Conference on Nutrition and Fitness. World Rev Nutr Diet. Basel, Karger, 1997, vol 81.
5 Simopoulos AP, Pavlou KN (eds): Volume II. Nutrition and Fitness: Metabolic and Behavioral Aspects in Health and Disease. Proceedings of the Third International Conference on Nutrition and Fitness. World Rev Nutr Diet. Basel, Karger, 1997, vol 82.

For further information contact:
Artemis P. Simopoulos, MD
Chairman, Third International Conference on Nutrition and Fitness
President, The Center for Genetics, Nutrition and Health
2001 S Street, NW, Suite 530
Washington, DC 20009 (USA)
Phone: (202) 462–5062
Fax: (202) 462–5241

Simopoulos AP (ed): Nutrition and Fitness: Evolutionary Aspects, Children's Health,
Programs and Policies. World Rev Nutr Diet. Basel, Karger, 1997, vol 81, pp 10–11

··························

Declaration of Olympia on Nutrition and Fitness

Ancient Olympia, Greece, May 26, 1992

- In developed countries technological developments have minimized physical activity, whereas variety and availability of foods make dietary choice a personal but not always well-advised decision.
- In most developing countries, the nutrition problems are quite different. Dietary fat is already low and unrefined carbohydrate high but the intake of energy, protein, and micronutrients are all too often inadequate. A more bountiful and sanitary supply of all the foods that are traditional in these cultures is needed. Surely, emulation of the excesses of the diets of Western affluent societies is to be avoided.
- The existence of large numbers of hungry children and adults amidst the abundance of food in many of the industrialized countries, is destructive to the individual and to society. Governments must correct the maldistribution problems that allow such inhumane inequities to exist and encourage food choices that provide optimal nutrition for all.
- The adverse health effects of physical inactivity and consumption of high-fat diets have been repeatedly demonstrated in affluent societies by the high incidence of chronic diseases associated with these factors.
- Programs encouraging physical activity and good nutrition have now been shown to reduce diseases associated with inactivity and ill-advised diets, and can promote the quality of life.
- Understanding of the benefits to health from increased physical activity and good nutrition should be widely disseminated through extensive publicity.
- Health professionals should be educated in nutrition and exercise physiology to assume leadership roles in educating the public to the health benefits of physical activity and good nutrition.

- Education of the public should be promoted in schools at all levels, in the work place, through the media, and by health professionals.
- Advice provided to the public should be based on validated research findings in nutrition, genetics, and physiology. Research in these interrelated biomedical sciences deserves increased public and private support.
- Communities must provide clean and open spaces for children's playgrounds and adults sports and designate specific paths for pedestrians, cyclists, and other exercisers.
- Evidence is now convincing that general well-being and health can be greatly advanced by achievable adjustments of life-styles, nutrition, and physical activity. We call on all to respond.

Simopoulos AP (ed): Nutrition and Fitness: Evolutionary Aspects, Children's Health,
Programs and Policies. World Rev Nutr Diet. Basel, Karger, 1997, vol 81, pp 12

....

Conference Resolutions

Ancient Olympia, Greece, May 26, 1988

At the completion of the conference the following resolutions were adopted unanimously:

(1) The participants of the conference wish to encourage governments to develop programs related to better nutrition and improved fitness.

(2) Nutrition policies should be coordinated with programs to improve physical fitness.

(3) Programs should take into consideration the variations in need in relation to different age groups and social circumstances for guidance about dietary needs and physical activity.

(4) IOC and WHO should be leaders in stimulating and providing guidance.

(5) We should meet in Olympia every 4 years before the Olympic games to update advice in the light of research results. We should continue to stimulate governments to develop and maintain programs on nutrition and fitness.

Simopoulos AP (ed): Nutrition and Fitness: Evolutionary Aspects, Children's Health,
Programs and Policies. World Rev Nutr Diet. Basel, Karger, 1997, vol 81, pp 13–23

....

Diet, Physical Activity, and Health: Policies for the New Millennium

Keynote Address

Philip R. Lee[a], Linda D. Meyers[b]

[a] Assistant Secretary for Health;
[b] Senior Nutrition Advisor, Office of Disease Prevention and Health Promotion,
United States Department of Health and Human Services, Office of Public Health
and Science, Washington, D.C. USA

Greece, a country that traditionally values quality of life, healthy lifestyles, and healthy families and children, is an especially fitting venue for this third International Conference on Nutrition and Fitness, a conference convened to consider two key determinants of health, diet and physical activity and dedicated to the concept of positive health. You will recall that it was a Greek, Hippocrates, who enunciated the concept of positive health and the interlinked nature of nutrition and physical activity and observed 'Eating alone will not keep a man well, he must also take exercise. For food and exercise, while possessing opposite qualities, yet work together to produce health' [1].

This conference emphasizes issues related to overconsumption of food and chronic diseases. We would be remiss, however, if we did not remember, as William Clay from the Food and Agriculture Organization noted so eloquently in his remarks [2], that undernutrition and issues of access to food are of paramount importance for many people in the world. Whether the focus is over- or underconsumption, our overall goal is the same: for all people, the ready availability of safe and nutritionally adequate foods, the ability to acquire acceptable foods, and the provision of an environment that encourages society to make nutrition and physical activity choices consistent with good health.

Over the past 40 years the senior author has worked in the public health arena as a clinician, academician, and government official, working first in international health and then domestic health policy. His present responsibilities include oversight of nutrition policy as well as physical acivity, fitness and sports within the United States Department of Health and Human Services (HHS). During the past 33 years he has been an active participant in the debates in the United States on diet and health and on physical activity and health. This paper draws on that unique perspective to discuss the evolution and implementation of dietary guidance policy in the United States, the emergence of physical activity as a key national priority, and the challenges inherent in effecting long-term lifestyle changes in diet and physical activity patterns.

Diet, Physical Activity, and Chronic Disease Prevention

During the past 40 years there has been a shift in diet-related public health problems from nutrient deficiency diseases as major problems to chronic degenerative diseases as leading causes of death. In 1995 four of the ten leading causes of death in the United States – heart disease, certain cancers, stroke, and diabetes mellitus – were diseases in which diet and physical activity play a role. Together these diseases account for nearly two-thirds of the more than two million annual deaths in this country [3]. If one counts alcohol as a dietary factor, the figure increases to 7 of the 10 leading causes of death [3]. This is because alcohol can be a contributing factor to deaths from unintentional injuries (especially those involving motor vehicles), suicides, homicides, and chronic liver disease and cirrhosis. Stated another way, dietary factors and activity patterns that are too sedentary together account for at least 300,000 deaths each year, second only to the 400,000 estimated for tobacco [4]. If excess consumption of alcohol is included, the figure increases to 400,000 deaths per year [4]. Sir Roger Bannister summarized the situation well when he stated at the first International Conference on Nutrition and Fitness that 'physical activity and nutrition are as important at the end of this century as plumbing, sanitation and increased food intake were at the beginning of the century' [5].

During the past decade, scientific consensus has emerged around dietary recommendations for disease prevention and health promotion. This consensus was brought to fruition in the 1988 Surgeon General's Report on Nutrition and Health [6] and the 1989 National Academy of Sciences report on Diet and Health: Implications for Reducing Chronic Disease Risk [7].

A similar consensus emerging around physical activity and health is expressed in the 1996 Surgeon General's Report on Physical Activity and Health [8]. More than a decade ago Stanford University's Paffenbarger and colleagues [9] summarized the state of science in their book Exercise and Health: The Evidence and the Implications. Their emphasis was on the benefits of aerobic exercise. In the last ten years, research has confirmed the benefits of aerobic exercise and has provided evidence of the benefits of regular physical activity, such as daily walking, for 30 minutes or more. In addition, evidence shows that exercises to increase strength, provide muscle stretching and promote balance all can add to overall well-being. Regular physical activity is good for all of us, but few engage in regular physical activity at the level needed for health benefits. In fact, more than 60% of adults are inactive or not active enough for health benefits [8]. What is not as well known but is becoming more evident is that inactivity is a major risk factor for many chronic diseases. It is not just that physical activity is good for us, but that inactivity is harmful.

Dietary Guidance Policy Development

The shift in emphasis toward chronic disease risk reduction is reflected in national policies. For example, Healthy People 2000, the national initiative for disease prevention and health promotion includes physical activity and fitness and nutrition as the first 2 of 22 priority areas [10].

Modifications in the dietary advice provided by the United States government illustrate the evolution of collective efforts to change lifestyle behaviors in the United States. In the early days of the century nutritional advice emphasized obtaining sufficient nutrients, including calories and fat, to avoid the nutrient deficiency diseases prevalent then. As the prevalence of nutrient deficiency diseases declined and such chronic diseases as heart disease and cancers became major public health problems, dietary guidance began to address the relationship between food components and these diseases, and on limiting some components, including calories and fat [11–13].

The first of this new type of guidance was issued in 1977 by the Senate Select Committee on Nutrition and Human Needs under the chairmanship of Senator George McGovern as the Dietary Goals for the United States [14]. That report for the first time recommended specific levels of nutrients to reduce risk for several chronic diseases, for example, less than 30% of calories from fat and less than 10% of calories from saturated fat. It also generated substantial controversy and discussion within the health and agricultural communities about the scientific basis and utility of its quantitative goals [15].

As a partial response, the Department of Health, Education, and Welfare (now Health and Human Services) asked the United States' American Society for Clinical Nutrition to form a panel to assess the scientific evidence on six dietary factors thought to be related to major chronic diseases. These were dietary cholesterol, saturated and unsaturated fat, carbohydrate and sucrose, alcohol, excess calories, and dietary sodium. The panel's findings, presented in 1979, were strongest for alcohol and liver disease, followed by carbohydrates

Table 1. Dietary Guidelines for Americans, 1980–1995

1980	1985	1990	1995
Eat a variety of foods	Eat a variety of foods	Eat a variety of foods	Eat a variety of foods
Maintain ideal weight	Maintain *desirable* weight	Maintain *healthy* weight	*Balance the food you eat with physical activity – maintain or improve your weight*
Avoid too much fat, saturated fat, and cholesterol	Avoid too much fat, saturated fat, and cholesterol	*Choose a diet low in* fat, saturated fat, and cholesterol	Choose a diet with plenty of *grain products, vegetables, and fruits*
Eat foods with adequate starch and fiber	Eat foods with adequate starch and fiber	*Choose a diet with plenty of vegetables, fruits, and grain products*	Choose a diet low in fat, saturated fat, and cholesterol (same but order changed)
Avoid too much sugar	Avoid too much sugar	*Use sugars only in moderation*	*Choose a diet moderate* in sugars
Avoid too much sodium	Avoid too much sodium	*Use salt and sodium only in moderation*	*Choose a diet moderate* in salt and sodium
If you drink alcohol, do so in moderation	If you drink *alcoholic beverages,* do so in moderation	If you drink alcoholic beverages, do so in moderation	If you drink alcoholic beverages, do so in moderation

Changes from previous edition are in italics; changes in text are not shown here.
Source: USDA and HHS. Nutrition and Your Health: Dietary Guidelines for Americans [18–20, 24].

and dental caries, salt and hypertension, cholesterol and fat, cholesterol, excess calories, and saturated fat [16]. These findings were reflected in the general recommendations in Healthy People: The Surgeon General's Report on Health Promotion and Disease Prevention [17].

The United States Department of Agriculture (USDA) and HHS also began to develop a set of simple guidelines that would provide guidance for people as they made daily food choices. The resulting guidelines and explanatory text were published in 1980 as Nutrition and Your Health: Dietary Guidelines for Americans [18]. The seven guidelines are shown in table 1. Although nonquantitative, these statements evoked considerable discussion by some nutrition scientists, consumer groups, commodity groups, the food industry, and others.

Later that year the United States Congress through the Senate Agriculture Appropriations Committee called for the Department of Agriculture to undertake a review of the *Dietary Guidelines* – clearly in response to concerns raised about it by beef and dairy industries. Thus, a Dietary Guidelines Advisory Committee of nine nutrition scientists was convened in 1983 to review and make recommendations to the two Departments about the guidelines. The Committee's recommendations for minor changes in the original guidelines were reviewed and slightly revised by government scientists, and the second edition of the *Guidelines* was published in 1985. The change of the term alcohol to alcoholic beverages and the term ideal to desirable in reference to weight were the only changes in the seven statements on the cover of the pamphlet, and even then the body weight table in the text remained unchanged [19]. In contrast to the first edition, the second edition was received with little controversy, likely a reflection of the growing body of research that supported the recommendations.

In keeping with their responsibilities to provide up-to-date advice about healthy dietary patterns to consumers, the Secretaries of HHS and USDA convened a second Dietary Guidelines Advisory Committee in 1989 to review the second edition, determine if revisions were warranted, and, if so, to recommend changes. This Committee had the benefit of the two major scientific reviews, the Surgeon General's Report on Nutrition and Health [6] and the National Academy of Sciences' report on Diet and Health: Implications for Reducing Chronic Disease Risk [7]. The Committee's report was issued in June 1990, revised slightly by the Departments, and the third edition released in November 1990 [20]. Again, the basic tenets of the original *Dietary Guidelines* were reaffirmed, and additional refinements specifically added in keeping with better understanding of the science of nutrition and how best to communicate that science to consumers. For example, quantitative upper limits on fat ($\leq 30\%$ calories from fat) and saturated fat ($< 10\%$ calories from saturated fat) were included for the first time in the explanatory text. In response to consumer evaluation studies, the guidelines were also stated more positively rather than as a dictum to 'avoid' [21].

Also in 1990, the United States Congress stipulated in the National Nutrition Monitoring and Related Research Act [22] that the *Dietary Guidelines for Americans* were to be published every five years jointly by HHS and USDA and were to be promoted in government nutrition-related programs, including the school lunch and breakfast programs. Thus, in a decade, the *Dietary Guidelines for Americans* had moved with only minor changes from a contentious document to one that provided the statutory basis of Federal nutrition education efforts.

The *Dietary Guidelines* review process was initiated again in 1994 [23, 24] and the 1995 edition was released by HHS Secretary Shalala and USDA Secretary Glickman on January 2, 1996 [25]. The seven guidelines themselves remain simple (table 1). They, along with the text that explains them, are collectively referred to as the *Dietary Guidelines for Americans* and constitute Federal dietary guidance policy. Once again, the basic principles of previous editions were reaffirmed, and there were changes that reflected emerging science [26]. One was the recognition of vegetarian diets as an alternative dietary choice. In addition, the *Guidelines*, which are applicable to all healthy persons 2 years of age and older, acknowledge that 'Eating is one of life's great pleasures', discourage weight gain with age for adults, encourage weight maintenance as a first step to achieving a healthy weight, provide specific guidance for children and dietary fat intake (gradual move to no more than 30% of calories from fat between the ages of 2 and 5), include a statement that moderate alcohol intake is associated with lower risk for coronary heart disease in some individuals, and highlight the Food Guide Pyramid and the new Nutrition Facts Label as key educational tools. Perhaps the biggest difference from the previous edition, however, is the renewed focus on health benefits of decreasing sedentary activity by increasing regular, moderate physical activity, including the recommendation for '30 minutes or more of moderate physical activity on most – preferably all – days of the week' and the specific inclusion of physical activity in the wording of the second statement on the cover [25].

Progress in Implementation

According to a recent comprehensive report of data on the nutritional status of Americans from the United States' National Nutrition Monitoring and Related Research Program, Americans are slowly changing their eating patterns towards more healthful diets [27]. A considerable gap remains, however, between public health recommendations and consumers' practices, whether dietary or physical activity. Illustrative 'snapshots' [8, 27–30] indicate that:

(1) Overweight is increasing. No matter how it is measured, more children, adolescents, and adults are overweight now than a decade ago.

(2) On the positive side, average intakes of cholesterol and of total fat and saturated fat as a percentage of calories, have decreased. For many Americans, however, they are still above recommended levels.

(3) The average daily intake of fruits and vegetables for the general population is about four servings. Fewer than one-third of adults meet the recommendation to consume five or more servings of fruits and vegetables per day.

(4) The examples go on. One striking example of changes in foods eaten has been the decline in whole milk consumption and the increase in nonfat milk consumption in adults. In children, however, one sees a decline in milk consumption and a more than compensating increase in soft drink consumption – a worrying trend.

(5) On the physical activity side, we know that almost one in four Americans is completely sedentary while over one half do little or no regular physical activity.

(6) Over 90% of older Americans do not exercise at levels sufficient to benefit heart health.

(7) While children are more active than adults, there is a dramatic decline in activity levels during adolescence.

(8) Only one of the 50 States now has a requirement for daily physical education in the schools for grades K-12.

Barriers and Strategies

While the observations above apply to the United States, they are similar to those in many industrialized countries [31], and we all need to be concerned with these patterns and the implications of their globalization, especially in view of the ready availability of higher calorie or fat or lower nutrient-dense foods worldwide. How can positive change be accelerated and negative patterns reversed? How can healthy diets and activity patterns become a routine part of daily lives? The overall environmental and lifestyle factors that impede adoption of healthy diets and physically active lifestyles are well recognized. In the United States, these include (1) the ubiquitous nature of television; (2) the constant barrage of quick fixes offering beauty, fancy cars, and a plethora of fast and fatty foods; (3) the increasing use of automobiles; (4) increased urbanization without safe space for walking, recreational activity or sports; (5) decreased allocations of funds for physical education in schools and grassroots sports in communties; (6) the lack of adequate health education, including nutrition education, in schools, and (7) increasing urban violence, just to name a few.

At the family and individual level, USDA data illustrate ways the recent changes in lifestyles affect eating habits – for example, many more people eat away from home – 50% on a given day [30]. By 1992, urban households spent more than one-third of their total food expenses on food away from home; by 1994 the number of women and young children eating away from home had increased by about 50% since the late 1970s [30].

Other barriers include failure to believe that chronic disease control can be affected by personal dietary choices and physical activity, lack of motivation and confusion about what specific actions to take, and ineffective changes (e.g. consuming less whole fat milk but more higher fat cheeses); and the many other roles of food and determinants of food choice in addition to health [32]. One often overlooked barrier to increased physical acitivity is cigarette smoking, which, along with its other debilitating effects, reduces the ability for one to be physically active; and smoking is on the increase among youth. In part this appears to be in response to the promotional efforts of the tobacco companies that convey the image of slimness and vigor associated with cigarette smoking.

To address these challenges will require concerted, creative, and consistent actions across public and private sectors. The following strategies, based on recent discussions among colleagues in follow-up to the International Conference on Nutrition [33], are put forth here for consideration and further enhancement.

- *Build multisectoral partnerships and commitment* to promote and maintain healthful dietary choices and physical activity.
- *Regularly update nutrition and physical activity program standards* to reflect current scientific consensus and government policy and to better prepare for ongoing and future changes in demographic trends, roles of men and women, norms of eating patterns, and demand by consumers for information.
- *Use state-of-the-art methods and technologies* to achieve behavioral change, including customer-oriented marketing techniques and new technologies. The Nutrition Facts label now required on all packaged foods in the United States is an example.
- *Expand proven interventions to fully reach target groups.* Interventions that have been shown to be effective and efficient in small scale studies and demonstrations need to be reviewed and tailored for various audiences with the goal of development, implementation, and evaluation of cost-effective interventions that reach all segments of the American public and promote adoption and maintenance of healthy dietary and physical activity patterns across the lifespan.
- *Improve school nutrition and physical education and activity programs of school-children* to help children develop healthy food and physical activity habits during formative years. Organized after school programs can also be very important, particularly to adolescents.
- *Increase the availability of food choices for a healthy diet in all types of commercial food service operations.* Restaurant, vending machine, and quick-stop grocery market consumers ought to demand, and food services operations need to provide and encourage choices consistent with the *Dietary Guidelines for Americans*, if they do not already do so.
- *Encourage increased physical activity in daily living* by fostering environmental changes such as safe and accessible stairs (with signs on elevators), safe and accessible walking and biking trails, parks, zoning restrictions that protect open spaces, and incentives that encourage physical activity and discourage physical inactivity.

- *Improve policy action through research and evaluation.* Research is needed to apply the new techniques of molecular biology to understand how dietary factors cause such profound ill consequences for health and to stimulate healthy food, nutrition, and physical activity behaviors. In addition, psychosocial research is needed on determinants of successful adoption and maintenance of physical activity and healthful dietary patterns and on the design, effective implementation, and evaluation of interventions to achieve long-term change.
- *Maintain a strong monitoring system* to track and evaluate physical activity, dietary and nutritional status changes and their determinants and consequences.

Conclusion

Our task is a challenging one, but one we have an obligation to continue. Dr. Abraham Horwitz, a global leader in nutrition, director emeritus of the Pan American Health Organization, and still active in his 80's, stated the challenge eloquently: 'Keep the faith that you are committed to a most noble cause, the well-being of people whom you do not know but whose needs you feel intensely. Redouble your efforts in whatever you do in nutrition (and, we would add, physical activity) while being bold and imaginative' [34]. Let us in our professional discussions and in our actions, be committed, bold and imaginative.

Acknowledgements

The authors thank Dr. Marion Nestle and Dr. Artemis Simopoulos for helpful comments and advice and Drs. Don Franks, York Onnen, and Christine Spain and Ms. Mary Ann Hill for useful, quick input during the development of this presentation.

References

1   Hippocrates: Regimen I. Translated by WHS Jones. Cambridge, Harvard University Press, 1953. Also reprinted in The Declaration of Olympia on Nutrition and Fitness, Ancient Olympia, May 26, 1992.
2   Clay W: Opening Remarks: Third International Conference on Nutrition and Fitness. Athens, Greece, May 1996.
3   Rosenberg HM, Ventura S, Mauer J, Heuser R, Freedman MA: Births and Deaths in the United States, 1995. Monthly Vital Statistics Report 1996;45(suppl):1–40.
4   McGinnis JM, Foege WH: Actual causes of death in the United States. JAMA 1996;270:2207–2212.

5   Bannister R Sir: Special presentation: Health, fitness and sport. Am J Clin Nutr 1989;49:927–930.
6   Department of Health and Human Services: The Surgeon General's Report on Nutrition and Health. Washington, USGPO, 1988.
7   National Research Council: Diet and Health: Implications for Reducing Chronic Disease Risk. Washington, National Academy Press, 1989.
8   US Department of Health and Human Services: The Surgeon General's Report on Physical Activity and Health. Washington, USGPO, 1996.
9   Thomas GS, Lee PR, Franks P, Paffenbarger RS: Exercise and Health: The Evidence and the Implications. Cambridge, Oelgeschlager, Gunn & Hain, 1981.
10 United States Department of Health and Human Services: Healthy People 2000: National Health Promotion and Disease Prevention Objectives. Washington, USGPO, 1990.
11 Nestle M, Lee PR, Baron RB: Nutrition Policy Update; in Weininger J, Briggs GM (eds): Nutrition Update, vol 1. New York, Wiley, 1983.
12 Nestle M, Porter DV: Evolution of federal dietary guidance policy: From food adequacy to chronic disease prevention. Caduceus 1990;6:43–87.
13 McGinnis JM, Nestle M: The Surgeon General's report on nutrition and health: Policy implications and implementation strategies. AM J Clin Nutr 1989;49:23–28.
14 Select Committee on Nutrition and Human Needs, United States Senate: Dietary goals for the United States, ed 2, Washinton, USGPO, 1977.
15 Simopoulos, AP: The scientific basis of the 'goals': What can be done now? JADA 1979;74:539–542.
16 Ahrens ED Jr, Connor WE, Bierman EL, Glueck CJ, Hirsch J, McGill HC, Spritz N, Tobian L, Van Itallie TB: Report of the task force on the evidence relating six dietary factors to the Nation's health. Am J Clin Nutr 1979;32:2621–2748.
17 US Department of Health and Human Services: Healthy People: The Surgeon General's Report on Disease Prevention and Health Promotion. Washington, USGPO, 1979.
18 US Department of Agriculture and US Department of Health and Human Services: Nutrition and Your Health: Dietary Guidelines for Americans. Washington, USGPO, 1980.
19 US Department of Agriculture and US Department of Health and Human Services: Nutrition and Your Health: Dietary Guidelines for Americans, ed 2. Washington, USGPO, 1985.
20 US Department of Agriculture and US Department of Health and Human Services: Nutrition and Your Health: Dietary Guidelines for Americans, ed 3. Washington, USGPO, 1990.
21 Dietary Guidelines Advisory Committee: Report of the Dietary Guidelines Advisory Committee on the Dietary Guidelines for Americans, 1990: To the Secretary of Health and Human Services and the Secretary of Agriculture. Beltsville, USDA/ARS, 1990.
22 US Congress: Public Law 101–445: National Nutrition Monitoring and Related Research Act of 1990. Washington, USGPO, 1990.
23 Bialostosky K, St. Jeor ST: The 1995 Dietary Guidelines for Americans. Nutr Today 1996;31:6–11.
24 Dietary Guidelines Advisory Committee: Report of the Dietary Guidelines Advisory Committee on the Dietary Guidelines for Americans, 1995: To the Secretary of Health and Human Services and the Secretary of Agriculture. Beltsville, USDA/ARS, 1995.
25 US Department of Agriculture and US Department of Health and Human Services: Nutrition and Your Health: Dietary Guidelines for Americans, ed 4. Washington, USGPO, 1995.
26 Kennedy E, Meyers L, Layden W: The 1995 dietary guidelines for Americans: An overview. JADA 1996;96:224–227.
27 Federation of Americans Societies for Experimental Biology, Life Sciences Research Office. Prepared for the Interagency Board for Nutrition Monitoring and Related Research: Third Report on Nutrition Monitoring in the United States (2 volumes). Washington, USGPO, 1995.
28 Kuczmarski RJ, Flegal KM, Campbell SM, Johnson CL: Increasing prevalence of overweight among US adults: The national health and nutrition examination surveys, 1960–1991. JAMA 1994;272:205–211.
29 Troiano RP, Flegal KM, Kuczmarski RJ, Campbell SM, Johnson CL: Overweight prevalence and trends for children and adolescents: The national health and nutrition examination surveys, 1963 to 1991. Arch Pediatr Adolesc Med 1995;149:1085–1091.

30 United States Department of Agriculture, Agriculture Research Service: What we eat in America 1994–1996: Results from the 1994 CSFII. Internet 1996.
31 International Conference on Nutrition: Nutrition and Development: A Global Assessment. Rome, FAO/WHO, 1992.
32 Frazao E: The American Diet: Health and Economic Consequences. Agriculture Information Bulletin 711. Washington, Economic Research Service, 1995.
33 United States Department of Agriculture, United States Department of Health and Human Services, United States Agency for International Development: Nutrition Action Themes for the United States: A Report in Response to the International Conference on Nutrition. Washington, USGPO, in press.
34 Horwitz A: Interview: Dr. A Horwitz, SCN Chair 1986–1995. SCN News 1995;13:1–3.

Philip R. Lee, MD, United States Department of Health and Human Services,
Office of Public Health and Science, 200 Independence Avenue, S.W.,
Suite 716–G, Washington, DC 20201 (USA)

Simopoulos AP (ed): Nutrition and Fitness: Evolutionary Aspects, Children's Health, Programs and Policies. World Rev Nutr Diet. Basel, Karger, 1997, vol 81, pp 24–25

....

Summary of Part 1

Artemis P. Simopoulos[a], *S. Boyd Eaton*[b]

[a] Center for Genetics, Nutrition and Health, Washington, D.C., and
[b] Emory University, Atlanta, Ga., USA

This first session consisted of five presentations. The speakers reviewed the evolutionary aspects of diet and exercise, the role of nutrients and exercise in gene expression, and the clinical studies underway.

Whereas man's genetic profile has not changed, major changes have taken place in both our dietary and physical activity patterns which appear to be responsible for the increase in chronic diseases, such as coronary artery disease, hypertension, diabetes, obesity, cancer, arthritis, and other autoimmune diseases, also known as diseases of civilization.

Eaton described the diet of ancestral humans. Compared with current nutrition, preagricultural humans consumed more fiber, protein, micronutrients (probably including phytochemicals), but less overall fat, less saturated fat and a more balanced n–6: n–3 ratio. Their foods were generally micronutrient rich, but energy dilute.

Phillipson related differences in the satiation effects of dietary fat and carbohydrate to the relative scarcity of fat in the diets of human ancestors extending millions of years into the past. She pointed out that while average life expectancy in classical times was brief, individuals who did live into their seventies and eighties were often exceptionally fit compared with similar-aged individuals in the present. She observed that 'neoteric' foods generally have a higher glycemic index than do foods consumed by humans before agriculture.

Cordain traced evolution of the human line over the past 7 million years showing that modern-day exercise requirements and capacities reflect selective pressures operating for our ancestors during that period. The activity patterns of hunter-gatherers most closely resemble those of preagricultural humans. For them, energy expenditure averages over 20 kcal/kg/day whereas, for sedentary office workers the average is less than 4.5 kcal/kg/day.

Simopoulos reviewed the evidence that both nutrients and physical activity influence gene expression and pointed out that exercise influences lipoprotein lipase gene expression which leads to beneficial metabolic changes such as a decrease in low-density lipoprotein cholesterol and triglycerides while increasing high-density lipoprotein. Similar effects are brought on by n–3 essential fatty acids. She referred to the previous papers, both of which described dietary changes leading to decreases in n–3 fatty acids and physical activity as contributing to increases in chronic diseases and the need to return to dietary and exercise patterns consistent with man's genetic profile. Simopoulos also emphasized that humans are storehouses of genetic diversity, hence overall health recommendations may not be appropriate for all individuals. For example, differences in apolipoprotein E (ApoE) levels affect response to dietary changes. She anticipates a new medical paradigm for the 21st century: (1) diagnostic DNA testing; (2) genotypically specific preventive recommendations, and (3) ongoing metabolic monitoring. She emphasized the critical functions of essential fatty acids of the polyunsaturated fatty acid (PUFA) family. They (1) affect membrane function; (2) influence platelet aggregation, and (3) most importantly, regulate nuclear events that govern gene transcription. In the 20th century, nutritional changes have unbalanced our PUFA supply, increasing n–6 and decreasing n–3 PUFA, while a sedentary life style contributes further to the development of chronic diseases.

Wilmore described the 'Heritage Family Study' which investigates the genetic basis for differences in response to exercise. The study protocol is well-designed and exceedingly detailed. While results are still preliminary, the emerging data suggest that genetic factors do affect (1) the degree of weight loss occurring with exercise, and (2) the rate of VO_{2max} improvement resulting from exercise.

Artemis P. Simopoulos, MD, The Center for Genetics, Nutrition and Health, 2001 S Street, NW, Suite 530, Washington, DC 20009 (USA)

Simopoulos AP (ed): Nutrition and Fitness: Evolutionary Aspects, Children's Health, Programs and Policies. World Rev Nutr Diet. Basel, Karger, 1997, vol 81, pp 26–37

....

Evolutionary Aspects of Diet: Old Genes, New Fuels

Nutritional Changes Since Agriculture

S. Boyd Eaton[a], *Loren Cordain*[b]

[a] Department of Radiology, Emory University School of Medicine and Department of Anthropology, Emory University, Atlanta, Ga.;
[b] Department of Exercise and Sport Science, Colorado State University, Fort Collins, Colo., USA

This paper contends that the nutritional patterns of current humans differ in important ways from those of our preagricultural human ancestors. The differences have serious implications for growth, development, and health, implications best appreciated in the light of three premises:

(1) Regarding susceptibility to chronic degenerative diseases, our current gene pool is hardly changed from that of Stone Age humans. The genetic constitution with which we are now endowed was selected through evolutionary experience for life circumstances which obtained in the past, not those which exist at present [1].

(2) Ancestral human nutrition was derived overwhelmingly from wild game and uncultivated plant foods. Depending on location, season and era, honey, fish and (in times of shortage) wild grains made varying contributions [2].

(3) Because they lacked motorized equipment, draft animals, and most simple machines, our ancestors' level of physical exertion greatly exceeded that at present; probably their caloric expenditure was about one-half more each day [3].

These premises lay the foundation for two propositions. First, we now eat substantially smaller amounts of the foods for which evolution has attuned our biochemistry and physiology. This is because we consume less energy overall, in line with our reduced physical exertion, and because we have developed and/or adopted a variety of new energy sources, foods which were not available (or at least little utilized) by human ancestors and which displace

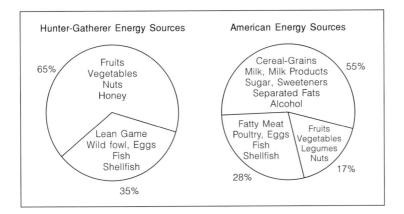

Fig. 1. Foods 'new' in evolutionary context have displaced/replaced a sizable fraction of the 'original' foods which fueled 99% of human evolution.

original, fundamental foods from our daily intake pattern (fig. 1). Second, the 'new' foods, which make up over half of what we now eat, include cereal grains, dairy products, prepared/processed foods, alcohol, separated fats, commercial meat, free salt, refined flours, and sweeteners. These collectively alter the mix of dietary constituents in ways detrimental to human health. That is, in addition to their passive effect of displacing much of the food which comprised nearly all Paleolithic human nutrition, the 'new' foods have an actively adverse influence resulting from constituents which have been shown to be harmful.

Nutrient Properties of Preagrarian Foods

Wild Vegetal Foods

The uncultivated fruits and vegetables consumed by hunters and gatherers generally contain high levels of micronutrients, except for sodium; potassium content greatly exceeds that of sodium in virtually all instances [2]. Some, such as nuts, beans, and seeds provide a substantial amount of fat, but this fat is predominantly unsaturated in nature and provides little of the C_{14}/C_{16} chain saturated fat which raises serum cholesterol levels [6]. Wild plants contain a considerable amount of dietary fiber, largely soluble in nature [7], which partly explains why their nutrient/food energy quotient is relatively great (table 1). The phytochemical content of wild plant foods is undetermined, but likely to be considerable, in line with their high average concentrations of vitamins and minerals [11].

Table 1. Energy and nutrients in vegetable foods

Food item(s) 100-gram portions	Energy kcal	Calcium, mg (mg/100 kcal)	Vitamin A, RE (RE/100 kcal)	Vitamin C, mg (mg/100 kcal)	Reference
Wheat, 5 varieties	331	39 (11.8)	0	0	8
Rice, brown	360	32 (8.9)	0	0	8
Granola	487	62 (12.7)	35 (7.2)	1 (0.2)	9
Pizza, cheese, no meat	245	155 (63.3)	132 (53.9)	5 (2.0)	10
French fries	275	15 (5.5)	tr.	22 (8.0)	10
236 uncultivated fruits/vegetables, mean	109	103 (94.5)	180 (165.1)	33 (30.3)	2

Wild Game

Game animals are typically lean, containing on average only one-fifth the fat and about half the energy provided by commercial meat. Game also has less cholesterol, but this difference is relatively slight. Fat from wild animals contains a high proportion (25–30%) of polyunsaturates, including the essential long chain constituents: arachidonic, eicosapentaenoic, and docosahexaenoic acids [6]. Because of its lower fat content, and hence lesser food energy, the nutrient/energy quotient of game, like that of wild plants, is high (table 2).

Nutrient Properties of Foods Introduced Since Agriculture

Cereal Grains

Wheat, rice, millet, corn and other grains made possible dramatic population growth as they became major dietary resources: they increased the total food energy which could be extracted from a given land area. But paleopathological findings at the origins of agriculture may in part reflect the nutrient/energy quotient of cereal grains which is lower than that of pre-agricultural foods (table 1). While whole grains are good fiber sources, especially for insoluble fiber, finely-milled flours contain hardly any fiber at all [7]. Cereals contain little fat of any type and especially little saturated fat; however polyunsaturated fat from certain commercially-important grains, including corn, is preponderantly omega-6 in nature [6]. Metaanalytic findings that grains have little cancer-preventive effect, relative to fruits/vegetables, suggest that their phytochemical content is lower and/or less effective.

Table 2. Energy and nutrients in animal foods

Food item(s) 100-gram portions	Energy kcal	Iron, mg (mg/100 kcal)	Thiamin, mg (mg/100 kcal)	Riboflavin, mg (mg/100 kcal)	Reference
T-bone Steak					
Total edible	397	2.2 (0.55)	0.06 (0.02)	0.13 (0.03)	8
Separable lean	164	3.2 (1.95)	0.09 (0.06)	0.19 (0.12)	8
Hamburger					
Regular	268	2.7 (1.01)	0.08 (0.03)	0.18 (0.07)	8
Lean	179	3.1 (1.70)	0.09 (0.06)	0.16 (0.09)	8
Frankfurters	309	1.9 (0.62)	0.16 (0.05)	0.20 (0.07)	8
Pork sausage	498	1.4 (0.28)	0.43 (0.09)	0.17 (0.03)	8
85 game species, mean	126	4.2 (3.33)	0.22 (0.18)	0.40 (0.32)	2

Dairy Foods

About half the energy in whole cow's milk is derived from fat, most of which is saturated. Furthermore, fat from dairy sources contains a substantial level of the C_{14}/C_{16} saturated fatty acids which raise serum cholesterol levels. Milk carbohydrate is all lactose, a simple sugar tolerated poorly by many humans. Cow's milk used for bottle feeding displaces the cellular macrophages and protein antibody immune factors previously supplied to infants from mothers' milk. Allergy to cow's milk proteins is a problem for a minority of the population and there is gradually increasing evidence that exposure to cow's milk protein during infancy and early childhood may promote development of type I diabetes mellitus in susceptible individuals [12].

Commercial Meat

During the late 19th and most of the 20th century, animals intended to provide meat were bred and raised to maximize their fat content; the much prized marbling effect and the price structure for prime, choice, and good beef, which vary stepwise in their fat content, are manifestations of this practice [6]. Thus, commercial meat animals have had, and still have to a lesser extent, a disproportionately high level of storage fat which is predominately saturated in nature and which contains a considerable amount of the C_{14}/C_{16} serum cholesterol-raising fatty acids. Compared with forage-fed animals, the polyunsaturated fat from grain-fed beef is skewed towards a high n–6:n–3 ratio [13].

Separated Fats

If they were like recently studied foragers, human ancestors eagerly sought fat, a desire reflecting its general scarcity in their diets coupled with the requirement for essential long-chain polyunsaturated fatty acids (PUFA). But preagricultural humans had no source of separated fat. Those now available vary in their nutritional effects, but all, including olive oil, make it possible to add gratuitous food energy to otherwise lower-fat containing foodstuffs, and frying emerged as a popular cooking technique only when separated fats became generally available [6]. Lard and dairy fats are sources of cholesterol-raising C_{14}/C_{16} saturated fatty acids while most vegetable oils provide a proportion of n–6 PUFA much higher than that of the fat typically available to ancestral humans [14].

Refined Flours and Sweetners

Perhaps reflecting the multi-million-year phase during which our remote primate ancestors were chiefly frugivorous, humans today like sweets. Hunter-gatherers enjoy honey to the point that in some localities and at favorable times of year it can provide 20% of total energy intake [15]. However, the relatively caries-free nature of most dental remains from the Paleolithic suggests that, in general, honey was much less available to our ancestors than are equivalent sweeteners today [16]. Both sweeteners and highly refined flours allow preparation of foods with artificially high energy content while they add few or no nutrients. Even refined flours fortified with vitamins and minerals lack the phytochemicals which appear to be constituents of fruits and vegetables.

Salt

Preagricultural humans, like a few isolated remaining current horticulturists, had no access to sodium except for that intrinsic to their basic foods. Nowadays, use of salt as a preservative, for food preparation, and as a seasoning has resulted in vastly increased human consumption: only 10% of the sodium consumed at present is intrinsic to our foods themselves [5]. This increased availability of sodium has inverted the sodium:potassium relationship which characterized human evolutionary experience. For human ancestors, as for other free-living terrestrial mammals, potassium intake greatly exceeded that of sodium; now this intake pattern is reversed [2].

Prepared and Processed Foods

Postagricultural humans are the only free-living mammals to consume foods whose natural origin is unrecognizable. Bread, cheese, sausage and similar items have been staples for millennia, but artificially fabricated foods have undergone an explosive increase in popularity during the past century. Food manufacturers were quick to recognize that salt, fat, and sugar were ingredients which enhanced acceptance of their products so a substantial proportion of the items in this general category provide empty calories, excessive fat, and often more sodium in a single serving than human ancestors obtained during a whole day [2].

Alcohol

Alcohol has been estimated to provide about 4.5% of average adult American energy intake [5]. Since most alcoholic beverages afford few if any nutrients, the energy derived from alcohol is another source of empty calories akin to sweeteners and highly refined flours. However, alcohol has pharmacological properties, some beneficial and some harmful, which distinguish it from other sources of food energy. Increasing evidence indicates that alcohol mitigates the development and/or consequences of coronary atherosclerosis [17], but it is associated with fetal alcohol syndrome, cirrhosis, accidents, violence, increased cancer risk, and chronic alcoholism [5]. No foragers studied in the past century have been able to make alcoholic beverages, so paleoanthropologists assume it was generally unavailable to preagricultural humans [18].

Old Foods vs. New Foods: Nutrient Implications

Energy

Until the late 19th century the circumstances of human existence appear to have demanded daily adult physical exertion which roughly equaled resting metabolic needs; that is, if resting metabolic rate (RMR) was 1,500 kcal/day, then total daily caloric expenditure was generally around 3,000 kcal [3]. This relationship seems to have characterized both Paleolithic and agricultural populations. However, in the late 20th century, the requirement for physical exertion, over RMR, has decreased by a staggering 60% or more [19]. For persons with an RMR of 1,500 kcal/day, typical total daily caloric expenditure is now 2,000 kcal or even less [3].

At the same time, the energy/nutrient quotient of our foods has increased. Commercial meat, separated fats, sweeteners, and many popular prepared/processed foods exhibit this property (tables 1, 2). In consequence, it is now possible to achieve (and often exceed) our energy needs, while our intake of nutrients other than energy is substantially lower than that which would be provided by 'natural' foods (i.e. ones consumed prior to agriculture). Nutrient intake is lower still in comparison to levels which would have been typical when activity patterns mandated greater energy intake. The latter point is not trivial: demand for essential nutrients increases with physical activity far less than the elevation in energy output would seem to warrant [20]. Thus, in the Paleolithic, when humans expended more energy through physical activity, the resulting increase in nutrient intake would have provided a reserve, or extra quota, above currently established requirements. This consideration may relate to contention regarding optimal and minimal nutrient levels [21].

Micronutrients

The immediately preceding discussion affects comparison of vitamin and mineral intake for Paleolithic and current humans. For such assessment it is most appropriate to contrast Stone Agers consuming 3,000 kcal/day with affluent Americans or Europeans eating only 2,000 kcal/day. If, for example, folate intake for an individual living 15,000 years ago was 0.136 mg/1,000 kcal and for a typical American 0.08 mg, then actual daily intake was likely to have been around 0.408 mg for the former and to be 0.16 mg for the latter. This makes the actual intake ratio 2.55 whereas simply comparing nutrients on the basis of dietary folate/1,000 kcal would suggest a deceptively lower ratio of 1.7 [2].

Any appraisal of preagricultural phytochemical intake must be purely speculative since, to the authors' knowledge, almost no determinations of such constituents have been made for uncultivated fruits and vegetables [but see ref. 11]. However, it seems likely that the phytochemical load for wild plants would have paralleled their high content of established micronutrients. Fruits and vegetables contributed a higher proportion of total energy for Stone Agers, typically about two-thirds of their intake as compared with roughly one-fifth to one-fourth for Europeans and Americans [2]. The foods we consume at present are often fortified with known vitamins and minerals, otherwise the discrepancy between Paleolithic and current micronutrient intake would be even greater than it is. However, phytochemical fortification is not practicable at present; therefore, the degree to which Paleolithic intake of such constituents exceeded our own was probably much more striking than the discrepancy in vitamin/mineral intake.

Electrolytes

Recently studied groups lacking free salt have electrolyte intake patterns reasonably similar to those retrojected for Paleolithic humans. Both populations consume(d) less than a gram of sodium and over five grams of potassium each day. In contrast, societies for whom salt is abundant commonly consume nearly 4 g of sodium, but only about 2,500 mg of potassium. All societies lacking salt have been found by anthropologists and/or epidemiologists to have low average blood pressures and virtually no hypertension [2, 18]; accordingly it is tempting to hypothesize that the control mechanisms regulating human blood pressure were selected during evolutionary adaptation to operate within a low-sodium, high-potassium nutritional context.

Fats

The relatively high fat content of dairy foods and commercial meat together with the availability of separated fat and the development of often high-fat prepared foods explain why fat intake in Western nations exceeds that for recently studied hunter-gatherers and, presumably, for preagricultural humans as well. Higher dietary fat content necessitates a greater overall energy/bulk ratio and thus, of itself, affects rates of obesity. However, changes in the nature of dietary fat are probably more important than is its increased contribution to total energy intake.

The fat available to contemporary humans is more highly saturated than that consumed by Stone Agers. The average content of C14 and C16 fatty acids in wild game is less than a fifth that found in commercial meat [6]. Highly saturated dairy fats were wholly unavailable to Paleolithic adults and, while coconuts, palm nuts and the like were locally available in certain geographical regions, their separated oils were not. Furthermore, commercially hydrogenated fats, which also raise serum cholesterol levels, are a recent innovation. These factors largely explain why foragers studied in this century, and who serve as inexact surrogates for Paleolithic humans, have serum cholesterol levels averaging around 125 mg/dl – despite dietary cholesterol intake well above 400 mg/day [6].

The ratio of n–6 to n–3 PUFA is estimated to have been far lower for preagricultural humans than for Americans [6, 14]. Game animals have considerably more n–3 PUFA relative to their n–6 PUFA content than do grain-fed commercial meat animals [13]. Because preagrarian humans ate so much wild game, their intake of n–3 PUFA from this source would have been considerable. In contrast, the vegetable oils currently used in the United States in prepared foods, for cooking, and as spreads afford far more n–6 than n–3 PUFA [14]. The ratio of dietary n–6 and n–3 essential fatty acids is thought to affect eicosanoid biosynthesis and thereby activity of n–6 and n–3 family eicosanoids [14, 22] so the higher level of n–6 PUFA relative to n–3 PUFA in current diets may have important physiological consequences.

Protein

The prominence of game in preagricultural economies insured that protein contributed a relatively greater proportion of overall energy intake for Stone Agers than at present. There must have been considerable variation depending chiefly on geographical location, but most paleoanthropologists believe that, on average, hunted and/or scavenged meat has provided about one-third of overall subsistence during the last 1.5 million years of human evolutionary experience [23]. This, in turn, suggests that protein (from both animal and vegetable sources) would have comprised 30–35% of daily energy for typical

Paleolithic humans. Even though their access to animal foods is far less, protein is estimated to provide from 1.6 to 5.9 g/kg/day for nonhuman primates. This compares with an estimated 2.5–3.5 g/kg/day for Stone Agers and contrasts with current recommendations of 0.8–1.6 g/kg/day [2].

Such high levels of dietary protein fit poorly with conventional nutrition theory. There is dispute as to whether high dietary protein adversely affects calcium balance, but its tendency to accelerate deterioration in renal failure is almost uncontested [24]. Regarding the latter, there is little evidence that high protein intake can, by itself, induce renal dysfunction and, since diabetes and hypertension were likely to have been rare, instances of kidney failure were presumably uncommon in the remote past.

There is, however, little reason to believe that such a high protein diet is 'necessary', at least with regard to nitrogen balance and maintenance of lean body mass, even in vigorously active individuals. For this reason possible protein-endocrine-eicosanoid relationships are intriguing [23]. The relative proportions of dietary protein and carbohydrate affect secretion of insulin and glucagon following a meal [25] and thereby influence both lipid metabolism and eicosanoid formation [26]. Integrated over the day, a higher proportion of protein to carbohydrate would act to increase the glucagon/insulin secretory ratio, thus reducing fat storage and inhibiting n–6 eicosanoid synthesis.

Fiber

Uncultivated vegetables and fruits tend to be highly fibrous so diets obtaining two-thirds of their energy from such sources necessarily provided a great deal of fiber, probably in excess of 100 g/day [7]. Both analysis of wild vegetal foods and evaluation of archaic native American coproliths support this estimate which is intermediate between nonhuman primate experience (for example, chimpanzees consume more than 200 g/day [2]) and dietary levels typical in affluent Western nations, which are generally below 20 g/day.

Like the high protein intake believed to characterize ancestral diets, daily fiber intake of 100 g or more fits ill with current concepts of optimal nutrition. Since the fiber consumed before agriculture was derived from fruits and vegetables rather than from grains, it provided little phytate, the factor of most significance relative to concerns about fiber's potentially adverse effect on mineral absorption. Furthermore, fruits and vegetables afford a higher proportion of soluble, fermentable fiber than do cereals, especially wheat and rice, whose fiber is preponderantly insoluble [7].

Formal, well-controlled evaluations of high-fiber diets in humans have focused on adults; however, the impact of such diets initiated after the conclusion of growth and development might differ from the effects of a similar diet consumed from childhood on. The latter, of course, more closely resembles the nutritional situation believed to have existed for preagricultural humans.

Discussion

Denis P. Burkitt wrote '... modern Western man has, in a very short period of time by evolutionary standards, deviated greatly from the biological environment to which his body has been adapted. This is the best explanation for ... the high frequency of Western diseases within the communities that have deviated most from the lifestyle of their ancestors ...' [27]. Similarly, James V. Neel believes '... there is now little room for argument with the proposal that health ... would be substantially improved by a diet and exercise schedule more like that under which we humans evolved' [1].

The endorsement of such respected figures is, of course, welcomed by proponents of paleonutrition, but well-designed, comprehensive research efforts directed towards testing its effects in current circumstances would be more desirable still. The core project would evaluate an experimental group consuming shellfish, lean meat, fish, vegetables and fruit – prepared and served without use of salt, separated fat, or oil. Dairy products and foods based on or containing cereal grains would also be excluded as would alcohol and sweeteners other than honey. In some studies individuals could self-select from the sanctioned food groups; others might employ a more structured dietary regimen, aiming to approximate the 30% protein, 45–50% carbohydrate, 20–25% fat pattern thought to be most representative of preagricultural experience. Because fruits, vegetables and lean meats available in affluent, industrialized nations differ nutritionally from their wild counterparts, the effects of supplementation to duplicate retrojected Paleolithic micronutrient levels and an n–6:n–3 ratio of 5 or less might be investigated as well. Further projects could explore the physiological and biochemical effects of paleonutrition in conjunction with typical Western sedentarism and compare the same nutritional protocol's influence on individuals exercising at or near Paleolithic levels. The program's effects on differing age groups might vary: older children, young adults, and aging individuals might benefit, or be harmed, to differing degrees.

Paleonutrition is an intellectually appealing, but unproved, dietary paradigm. Its theoretical basis is arguably more logical than vegetarianism and the Mediterranean or East Asian nutritional models. However, the latter have been formally investigated; each has benefits and drawbacks, while for paleonutrition similar advantages and flaws have not been determined. It is possible that life circumstances prevailing in affluent industrialized nations, including longer life expectancy, may interact adversely with the dietary (and physical exertion) patterns which prevailed while our gene pool was being selected. Alternatively, the insights of Neel and Burkitt may be correct. In either case, the ancestral human pattern, in force during nearly all the two million year experience of humanity, deserves serious investigation by current nutrition scientists.

References

1   Neel JV: Physician to the Gene Pool. New York, Wiley, 1994, pp 302, 315, 355.
2   Eaton SB, Konner, MJ, Shostak M: An evolutionary perspective enhances understanding of human nutritional requirements. J Nutr 1996;126:1732–1740.
3   Cordain L, Gotshall RW, Eaton SB: Health and fitness aspects of exercise: An evolutionary perspective. Int J Spts Sci 1997; in press.
4   Lee RB: What hunters do for a living, or how to make out on scarce resources; in Lee RB, DeVore I (eds): Man the Hunter. Chicago, Aldine, 1968, pp 30–48.
5   Food & Nutrition Board, Committee on Diet and Health, National Research Council. Diet and Health. Washington, National Academy Press, 1989, vol 55, pp 414, 436.
6   Eaton SB: Humans, lipids, and evolution. Lipids 1992;27:814–820.
7   Eaton SB: Fibre intake in prehistoric times; in Leeds AR (ed): Dietary Fibre Perspectives: Reviews and Bibliography. 2. London, Libbey, 1990, pp 27–40.
8   Watt BK, Merrill AL: Composition of foods. Agriculture handbook No. 8. Washington, US Department of Agriculture, 1963, pp 12, 15, 52, 55, 66.
9   Douglass JS, Matthews RH, Hepburn FN: Composition of foods. Breakfast cereals. Agriculture Handbook No. 8–8. Washington, US Department of Agriculture, 1982, p 53.
10 Leveille GA, Zabik ME, Morgan KJ: Nutrients in Foods. Cambridge, The Nutrition Guild, 1983, pp 172, 202, 208.
11 Simopoulos AP, Norman MHA, Gillaspy JE, Duke JA: Common purslane: A source of omega-3 fatty acids and antioxidants. J Am Coll Nutr 1992;11:374–382.
12 Karjalainen J, Martin JM, Knip M, et al: A bovine albumin peptide as a possible trigger of insulin-dependent diabetes mellitus. N Engl J Med 1992;327:302–307.
13 Marmer WN, Maxwell RJ, Williams JE: Effects of dietary regimen and tissue site on bovine fatty acid profiles. J Anim Sci 1984;59:109–121.
14 Kinsella JE, Broughton KS, Whelan JW: Dietary unsaturated fatty acids: Interactions and possible needs in relation to eicosanoid synthesis. J Nutr Biochemistry 1990;1:123–141.
15 Hill K, Hurtado AM: Hunter-gatherers of the new world. Am Scient 1989;77:437–443.
16 Smith P, Prokopec M, Pretty G: Dentition of a prehistoric population from Roonka Flat, South Australia. Arch Oceania 1988;23:31–36.
17 Marmot M, Brunner E: Alcohol and cardiovascular disease: The status of the U-shaped curve. Br Med J 1991;303:565–568.
18 Eaton SB, Konner M, Shostak M: Stone agers in the fast lane: Chronic degenerative diseases in evolutionary perspective. Am J Med 1988;84:739–749.
19 National Food Survey Committee: Household Food Consumption and Expenditure, 1990. London, HMSO, 1995, pp 55–114.
20 Astrand P-O: Whole body metabolism; in Horton ES, Terjung RL (eds): Exercise, Nutrition, and Energy Metabolism. New York, Macmillan, 1988, pp 1–8.
21 Rosenberg IH: Nutrient requirement for optimal health: What does that mean? J Nutr 1994;124: 1777S–1779S.
22 Sears B: Essential fatty acids and dietary endocrinology: A hypothesis for cardiovascular treatment. J Adv Med 1993;6:211–224.

23   Eaton SB, Konner M: Paleolithic nutrition: A consideration of its nature and current implications. N Engl J Med 1985;312:283–289.
24   Pedrini MT, Levey AS, Lau J, Chalmers TC, Wang PH: The effect of dietary protein restriction on the progression of diabetic and nondiabetic renal diseases: A meta-analysis. Ann Intern Med 1996; 124:627–632.
25   Westphal SA, Gannon MC, Nuttall FQ: Metabolic response to glucose injested with various amounts of protein. Am J Clin Nutr 1990;52:267–272.
26   Brenner RR, Nutritional and hormonal factors influencing desaturation of essential fatty acids. Prog Lipid Res 1981;20:41–47.
27   Burkitt DP, Eaton SB: Putting the wrong fuel in the tank. Nutrition 1989;5:189–191.

Dr. S.B. Eaton, Department of Radiology, West Paces Medical Center,
3200 Howell Mill Road, N.W., Atlanta, GA 30327 (USA)

Simopoulos AP (ed): Nutrition and Fitness: Evolutionary Aspects, Children's Health, Programs and Policies. World Rev Nutr Diet. Basel, Karger, 1997, vol 81, pp 38–48

Paleonutrition and Modern Nutrition

Connie Phillipson

Institute of Paleonutrition Studies, Athens, Greece

Scientists have come to nutrition from a variety of disciplines ranging from medicine to genetics, to molecular biology. I come from archeology and paleonutrition. And my special field is what I call 'evolutionary nutrition'. This is the study of the changing human foods and eating habits from the viewpoint of our genes and physiological conditioning; how biological and social evolution of our species have affected both our foods and dietary habits, and inevitably also our health and disease patterns.

Evolutionary nutrition encourages the study of questions that begin with 'why'. Here I have chosen to ask *and* answer 3 typical questions representing three different periods of the human past, to give you a first idea of the scope of evolutionary nutrition.

Effect of Carbohydrate and Fat on Human Appetite

The first question concerns the now well-known fact that carbohydrate and fat do not have the same effect on human appetite. A carbohydrate supplement at breakfast suppresses the appetite as measured an hour and a half later. By contrast, the same amount of energy in the form of fat has no such effect on appetite [1]. Considering that humans have carohydrate reserves for a maximum of 1 day, but fat reserves for 70 days [2], this satiety control for carbohydrate intake but its absence for fats, strikes one as unusually bizarre. One could perhaps readily understand the reverse situation, that is a satiety mechanism for fat and its absence for the plant fuel. As things stand, an obvious question appears to formulate itself here.

There is no oddity in the light of evoltionary nutrition. The disproportionately weak action of fat in satisfying the appetite may well be due to the importance of fats as an energy source, and the limited amount of fats in our hunter ancestors' diets.

There is no doubt at all that fat is the most efficient and economical natural storage of energy in existence. For one, fat packs more than twice the calories of carbohydrate and protein per unit weight [3]. For another, fat is stored by itself at a cost of only 3% of the energy stored. By contrast glycogen, the carbohydrate energy reserve, is stored with 3–4 parts of water at a cost of 23% of the stored energy [4].

But our hunter ancestors obtained relatively small amounts of fat from their diet. The flesh of most animals they hunted had less than 4% fat, instead of 20% in our meat, and there were very few other sources of fat in their diet [5].

In such circumstances there was no reason for our organism to develop for fat, a similar, powerful satiating action as it has for carbohydrates. Plant foods were easily available and the body had to be protected from excesses. Fat was not. As late as the 1960s, Nigerians ingested an average of only 6% fat, despite the easy availability of palm oil on the coastal areas of Nigeria. This was only half that of Japanese, who have one of the leanest diets on record. So for some populations of this earth, a satiating action for fat would have served no purpose as late as the middle of this century.

This applies with far greater rigor in the life of hunters, irrespective of whether the hunt takes place in the Kalahari Desert, or the Arctic. Even today the Kalahari Bushmen sometimes have to follow the wounded game for 2 days before it drops from exhaustion, even though the hunter's glycogen stores would barely last 24 h [6]. The long, low-intensity chase is precisely the condition when the preferred fuel of the organism is fat [7], when the hunter could spare no time to seek the plant foods to replenish his glycogen stores. Bushmen hunter-foragers carry this fat where it would do the least damage: their buttocks. This is a condition known as steatopygia, or fat rump, which is a Late Paleolithic feature of hunting populations confirmed from their mobiliary art [8].

For the Arctic Eskimos, fat may be even more important. In the cold temperatures where the hunt takes place, thermoregulation is of the utmost importance, not only for the hunt but for survival itself, and large energy reserves a stark necessity. But for this condition too, fat is the most effective fuel, and Inuit hunters eat more than 2,000 kcal a day in the form of fat [9]. So, the different satiation effects of carbohydrates and fats is no accidental coincidence, but the combination of two powerful realities: the hunter's need for large energy reserves, and the fact that fat is the most efficient energy storage. In short, fat is a hunter's fuel. This is as true of humans as of aquatic hunting mammals like seals and dolphins: thermoregulation demands their large fat stores. By contrast, fish with much smaller fat reserves adapt their body temperature to that of the water, while at the same time limiting their activities to essentials only.

Evidence of Tryptophan

Striking confirmation of the importance of fat comes from the metabolism of the essential amino acid tryptophan, which is the predecessor of serotonin, a neurotransmitter and appetite suppressant. It is well known that a carbohydrate meal raises tryptophan, both in the blood and in the brain. The extra brain tryptophan is usually explained by the rise of glucose, causing higher insulin secretions, and these in turn raising tryptophan in the brain. Tryptophan activates the brain's satiety mechanisms when it is metabolized to serotonin [10].

However, the addition of protein to a carbohydrate meal raises again the tryptophan in the blood, but *not* in the brain. Something that's quite incomprehensible, for it is known that the addition of protein to a carbohydrate meal lowers the plasma glucose, but often sharply raises its insulin [11, 12; see ref. 24]. Therefore, if raised blood insulin is responsible for the extra brain tryptophan, this should be even higher after a mixed meal, not lower. Needless to say, this fact remains without an explanation.

For evolutionary nutrition, the explanation is straightforward. The mixed meal is understood by the body as a time of plenty; a time to store fuel in its most economical form: fat. The extra insulin derived from mixed meals blocks the breakdown of fat and causes the deposition of more. A still unknown, but probably genetically controlled mechanism blocks the production of extra brain tryptophan and ensuing serotonin, despite the high blood insulin, to ensure that the satiety mechanism remains inactive and the appetite going. That, for the same reason our bodies have no satiety mechanisms for fat – what is a hunter's ideal fuel.

Evidence of the Human Kidney

The importance of animal protein and its complement of fat in the life of hunters is not attested only in metabolic processes like erratically high insulin secretions and the odd behavior of tryptophan accompanying mixed meals; it is also testified in some of our internal organs. It is already known that our kidneys possess a far greater filtering capacity than necessary. This is shown by the number of extra glomeruli found in the outer part or cortex of the kidney, usually at a resting state. These become active only when hyperfiltration is needed. That is, when large amounts of meat are eaten during a meal, and a greater capacity for the excretion of urea and the conservation of fluids and electrolytes is required [13].

But this kind of meal took place occasionally when a kill was made, and certainly not everyday, let alone more than once a day. Typically, hunters have no kidney disease despite their, from time to time, large protein intake. Just as typically, their more civilized descendants have several kinds of kidney disorders, and more than 8 million Americans suffer from them [14]. This is because the extra capacity of the kidney is used everyday, instead of on occasion only as it was designed. Renal disease in the West is inexorably progressive, because of 'a fundamental mismatch between the evolutionary design of our kidneys and the functional burden we place on them by our modern eating habits' [13].

Implications of Average Longevity

The second question concerns the frequent contention that many ancient populations had very brief life spans. Thus, estimates of the average longevity in ancient Greece and Rome range from 20 to 30 years [15], implying that contemporary Western society with its acknowledged much longer life span must be a lot healthier, or at least more vigorous.

However, studies based on average longevity, or life expectancy at birth, are subject to basic confounding variables; such as the distortion introduced by infant mortality, or the less well-known bias of death statistics. Dental and bone evidence may often be reliable. But some infectious diseases, epidemics, poisoning, and wounds to the skin, muscles, and internal organs are not amenable to the usual paleopathological investigation [16]. Death statistics may be very misleading [17], and there is considerable historical evidence that clearly contradicts the implications of the short life span at birth.

The ancient Greeks considered that a man reached his peak at the age of forty [18]. Aristotle advised men not to marry before the age of 35. This is hardly indicative of a short life span or a generally enfeebled middle age; but then neither are the lives and actions of Greeks whose age at death we happen to know, like many generals of Alexander the Great, for example. Antigonos Monophthalmos was a one-eyed Governor of Phrygia during a part of Alexander's campaigns. His imposing size and single eye induced his ever devoted soldiers to affectionately and mockingly call him 'the Cyclope'. An older general, he had served Alexander's father Philip in many battles. He usually took part in these mounted on his horse from where he indulged in restrained banter, casual jokes, and sometimes in liberal abuse towards his enemies. He was killed fighting in the Battle of Ipsus in 301 BC, overwhelmed by a cloud of javelins. He was 81 years old at the time. His main opponent and victor was Lysimachos, another one of Alexander's generals and the first

Hellenistic king of Thrace. He was defeated and killed fighting at the Battle of Corupedium in 281 BC. He was then 79 years old. His victor was his former ally in the Battle of Ipsus, Selefcos Nicator, the first Hellenistic king of Syria. Invading Europe just 1 year after Lysimachos's death, he was assassinated when he was 78 [19]. Surely these are remarkable ages for men to be wielding the heavy weapons of the period.

We may yet achieve a greater longevity in our own times, of course. But, as Alexis Carel wrote earlier this century, longevity is desirable when it prolongs youth, not old age. With a Mediterranean diet as everyday fare, an appetizing and popular fatty fish sauce called *gharos* rich in n–3 fatty acids, and a lot more exercise than is customary in our society, the ancient Greeks seem to have known both the secret of longevity and that of prolonging youth well into old age [20].

Historical as all this evidence is, however, it is also largely anecdotal. It is no substitute for the controlled clinical trial or intervention study that alone can give quantitative results. As it happens such a study was recently published.

Benefits of the Cretan Diet

An intervention trial involving 605 patients recovering from myocardial infarction was carried out by Serge Renaud and his co-workers. Its aim was to compare the prudent diet of the American Heart Association, with an adaptation of the Cretan diet [21]. After an average follow-up period of 27 months, recurrent myocardial infarction, all cardiovascular events, and cardiac and total deaths were reduced by over 70% in the group consuming the Cretan Mediterranean diet, what can only be called a highly significant result.

The protective effects were not related as one may expect to plasma total, LDL or HDL cholesterol, but rather to plasma fatty acids. That is, an increase of n–3 fatty acids and oleic acid and a decrease in linoleic acid. All these resulted from higher intake of linolenic and oleic acids and lower intake of saturated fats and linoleic acid from polyunsaturated fats.

The conclusion of this intervention trial is that the Cretan Mediterranean diet adapted to a Western population, protected against coronary heart disease much more efficiently than the diet of the American Heart Association. This was already suggested, of course, by the work of Keys and colleagues in the Seven Countries Study [22], but these were epidemiological findings and as such subject to all the confounding variables of such studies. An intervention trial with these results, on the other hand, has a very different bearing on the subject.

All this shows that there is more to the anecdotal evidence mentioned previously, showing men in their late seventies and eighties wielding weapons and fighting battles fit only for much younger men in our society. The no doubt simultaneous high rate of infant mortality, infectious disease, or other uncontrollable variables, should not be allowed to confuse the issue, nor hide their relative freedom from chronic degenerative disease for that matter, except for the ever-present degenerative spondylitis, which need not have interfered with everyday pursuits [23].

Glycemic Index

The third question I will touch upon is contemporary and concerns the higher glycemic index of what I call 'neoteric foods' for want of a better name. The glycemic index is a physiological measure of the glucose released by foods, as compared to the ingestion of an equal amount of glucose [24]. By neoteric foods I mean new, natural foods for the human stomach, not fast foods, junk foods or genetically modified foods. The case of the potato as such a food is well known. Roots as a group have a high average glycemic index of 72. But cooked potatoes can even surpass pure glucose with a glycemic index of 100 [25]. By contrast, sweet potatoes and taro from SE Asia and yams from Africa, demonstrably much older foods for Western stomachs, have much lower glycemic indices of 49, 54 and 51, respectively [26].

One could conclude from this that new foods have higher glycemic indices than older, more familiar, and equivalent foods. That would make sense from the viewpoint of evolutionary nutrition, but this does not quite fit vegetables like carrots and parsnips, which have high glycemic indices but are *not* new foods for the Western stomach. Both carrots and parsnips are well known from prehistoric Swiss lake-dwellings going back more than 6,000 years [27]. They are both known to be indigenous to Europe, so they hardly qualify as new foods, something which also warns against rushing to generalizations.

However, an interesting detail casts a somewhat different light on the subject. Carrot in its wild form has a woody and wiry root that is not very inviting. It responds rapidly to cultivation with great improvement in quality and appears to have been cultivated in the Mediterranean area during several centuries BC. Its presence in the wild form probably induced the early use of its leaves as a herb only. Thus, though it has been recognized in the garden of the Babylonian King Marduk II, the Biblical King Merodach-Baladan of the 8th century BC [28], it is placed among the scented herbs together with fennel, which suggests that the root was disregarded. Certainly, the carrot as root did not acquire importance as a food until quite late [27, p 111].

The history of the parsnip is obscured by the confusion of various names the Romans used for similar root vegetables. But Columella, the Roman writer of the 1st century AD, says that the unopened flowers of this plant were collected and stored as herbs, even though the root vegetable is known to have been imported from Germany for the table of the Roman Emperor Tiberius of the first century AD [27, p 112] and perhaps for other aristocrats.

Therefore, it seems quite possible that our ancestors used many vegetables indigenous to their lands, but in the beginning they ate only the leaves or flowers. Of these same vegetables we eat the roots, which are very different foods, with vastly different glycemic indices and metabolic processing. When we maintain that we eat the same foods as our ancestors, we must be fairly sure that we also eat the same parts of that food as they did.

Unfortunately, we still have a long way to go before we can understand fully what these changes meant for human intermediate metabolism. Thus, for example, we still do not know what is the glycemic index of potatoes for the people living on the Peruvian altiplano, where potatoes were first cultivated thousands of years ago. The same is true about maize for the inhabitants of Southern Mexico, and so on.

Yet it may be important to know the difference in the glycemic index of foods native to some lands, later introduced to others, together with the earliest dates when these foods were first eaten as may be gathered from excavations. This may give us some valuable quantitative clues about the influence of foods on our genes, what our physiological absorption rates are, how they change with food familiarity, and perhaps some other important metabolic processes that we do not quite understand yet.

A Dietary Basis for Manic Behavior?

I would like to end with a question that you would not normally hear from a nutritionist. Have you ever wondered why the cult followers of the god Dionysos, the Maenads, widely known from ancient Greek tragedy for their wild and unruly behavior, were largely confined to the area of Boeotia of central Greece?

I have often wondered whether there is a dietary connection with the strange behaviour of the Maenads. It is suspected that high intake of the trace element vanadium is associated with a manic state and other mental disorders. This is confirmed by the elevated blood and hair vanadium of manic patients. When this is reduced by a low vanadium diet or the administration of vitamin C to remove the excess, the condition markedly improves [29].

Manic behavior in antiquity was associated with the worship of the god Dionysos, better known perhaps under the name of Bacchus. The worship of Dionysos was celebrated in many ancient plays by Aeschylus, such as *Edonoi, Bassarides, Xantriae* and *Pentheus,* all unfortunately lost. The classic surviving depiction of Dionysiac worship and ecstasy is the play of Euripides, *Bacchae.*

In ancient Greece the women of Thebes, the largest Boeotian city, followed Dionysos to the mountains of Boeotia and became his Maenads. There they hunted animals and devoured their flesh and entrails raw, in what Egon Friedell called the 'epidemic psychoses' of the wildly orgiastic worshippers of the god, 'beyond all human concerns, conventions and fears' [30].

The question is what evidence is there for a source of vanadium in Boeotia? Well, typically vanadium occurs in igneous rocks. Vanadium is also known to occur in most bauxites [31]. Boeotia and neighboring states contain a fairly large number of bauxite deposits formed from larger serpentinite bodies. The weathering of these ultrabasic rocks might have given rise to the high vanadium in bauxites, but also to a soil with a good vanadium content. Some plants of the Astragalus species are vanadium accumulators, and *Astragalus bisulcatus* is a universal indicator of vanadium [32]. But do such plants grow in Boeotia? Indeed they do, and two species have been named accordingly: *Astragalus boeoticus* and *Astragalus parnassi*.

Even more to the point, of the five kinds of radishes known to Theophrastus, the sweetest was the Boeotian variety. It was widely cultivated and known as a cheap relish [33]. Radishes are a favorite food of rabbits, hares and other digging animals [34]. As it happens, with the exception of parsley and lobster, radishes contain the largest amount of vanadium of all other foods. A mere 100 g of radishes contain 790 µg of vanadium. This is 3–7 times the average daily human intake of the metal [35]. By contrast, the same quantity of potatoes has only 1 µg of vanadium.

As a metal, vanadium would have been concentrated in the liver and other internal organs of animals feeding on plants growing on rich vanadium soil. Naturally, the bioavailability of concentrated metals is much greater from animal sources, particularly so from their internal organs.

This kind of vanadium absorption could have easily predisposed some innocent consumers in Boeotia, who were more susceptible to ritual, to perhaps more frantic or unbalanced behavior. In North America some species of Astragalus are called loco weeds, because animals feeding on them act as if they are crazy (Spanish; loco) [36].

Only all this is a little theoretical. One may justly wonder if there are such high vanadium bauxites in the area. Well, the average vanadium content of bauxites is more than 18 times the mean of the unaltered rocks [37].

How realistic is such an assessment? One frankly wonders. It is probably as realistic as saying that modern Western society is less mentally balanced than that of our ancestors, partly because many tanks used by the food industry to process foods under pressure, are made out of high vanadium steel [35]. Although the evidence is anecdotal, I venture to submit it to your thoughtful inquiries and audit, since processed foods are not yet the objects of paleonutrition studies.

Conclusions

I hope to have managed in this brief paper to give you an idea of the benefits which paleonutrition, and especially evolutionary nutrition, can bring to modern nutrition and fitness by asking appropriate questions; and using the historical, archeological and other evidence available mainly from the physical sciences to try and answer them. Of course, questions which begin with 'why' are not very popular except in theoretical science, since they invariably demand mental excursions outside one's specialty. But the many 'whens' and 'hows' we have succeeded in answering during our technological revolution have not prevented the deterioration of human health to the point that in the US at least, public health spending is the major obstacle to balancing the budget – something that as late as the 1960s would have seemed simply inconceivable. What is happening in the Third World is by all accounts even worse, even though no one there has the temerity to think of balanced budgets.

It is perhaps time to revise our convictions once more and remind ourselves that in scientific endeavors clear thinking is not the result of formulas but the other way around: formulas are the result of processual thinking. If this process is inherently risky and full of hidden traps, the formula is no less so. It is almost established tradition that some of science's most cherished theories have furnished posterity's favorite chuckles. Adhering to formulas is no guarantee of diligence or of long-term immunity from scathing criticism. In the long run, it may be less harmful to try and be found wrong, than not to try out of fear of not being right. Or in the more poetic words of Cherteton, it would be a pity to admit that the process has not been tried and found wanting, but found difficult and left untried. It is in this spirit that we are trying to establish an Institute of Paleonutrition in Athens, Greece, and Nairobi, Kenya, for the obvious advantages such locations can give to the researcher in paleonutrition.

Recommendations

Many peculiar and until now unexplained effects known from nutrition research, cast unexpected light on human metabolic processes when examined from the viewpoint of evolutionary nutrition. They appear to confirm the primary role which the earlier eating and living habits of our species had on our genetic code. It seems reasonable to think that more work along these lines may help further clarify many of the metabolic processes which are so vital for our welfare.

Older diets such as the Cretan diet or other traditional Mediterranean diets are now known to be highly protective against modern chronic degenerative diseases like hypoglycemia, diabetes, hypertension, heart disease, obesity, and some forms of cancer. The fact is, however, that the healthy lifestyle of these people was not the outcome of some profound molecule-by-molecule understanding or an adherence to nutrition principles, but the result of a much simpler truth. They consumed their traditional foods mainly because these were the only ones they could afford. When greater wealth made it possible, these same people have largely opted for a more Westernized diet, with predictably adverse results. This may indicate that perhaps more emphasis on traditional foods may be more successful in turning more of the general public towards healthier eating habits, than the current practice of counting nutrients and calories.

Finally, neoteric foods may have higher glycemic indices than traditional foods, but they also present an opportunity to study the effect of new foods on human metabolism in ways that would be otherwise impossible in a species with such a long life span. It should not be difficult to determine the glycemic indices of such foods in people who have eaten them for several millennia, and it would be significant to know of any existing differences.

References

1 Blundell JE, Burley VJ, Cotton JR, Lawton CL: Dietary fat and the control of energy intake: Evaluating the effects of fat on meal size and postmeal satiety. Am J Clin Nutr 1993;57(suppl): 772S–778S.
2 Garrow JS: Energy balance and weight regulation; in Garrow JS, James WPT (eds): Human Nutrition and Dietetics. Edinburgh, Churchill-Livingstone, 1993, pp 137–145.
3 McNeill G: Energy; in Garrow JS, James WPT (eds): Human Nutrition and Dietetics. Edinburgh, Churchill-Livingstone, 1993, p 27, table 3.3.
4 Shah M, McGovern P, French S, Baxter J: Comparison of a low-fat, ad libitum complex-carohydrate diet with low-energy diet in moderately obese women. Am J Clin Nutr 1994;59:980–984.
5 Eaton SB, Konner M: Paleolithic nutrition. N Engl J Med 1995;312:283–289.
6 Westerterp KR: Food quotient, respiratory quoteint, and energy balance. Am J Clin Nutr 1993; 57(suppl):759S–765S, esp 760S, table 1.
7 Newsholme EA, Calder P, Yaqoob P: The regulatory, informational, and immunomodulatory role of fat fuels. Am J Clin Nutr 1993;57(suppl):738S–751S.
8 For an interesting comparison between the Bushman fat-rump and Paleolithic Venus figurines, see Bishop CW, Abbott CG, Hrdlicka A: Man From the Farthest Past. New York, Smithsonian Scientific Series 7, 1930, p 80, fig 16.
9 Eskimos may consume as much as 80 percent of their energy intake as fat; see Gurr M: Fats; in Garrow JS, James WPT (eds): Human Nutrition and Dietetics. Edinburgh, Churchill-Livingstone, 1993, pp 77–102, esp 87.
10 Wright JV: Dr Wright's Guide to Healing Nutrition. New Canaan, Keats, 1990, p 282.
11 Chew I, Brand JC, Thorburn AW, Truswell AS: Applications of the glycemic index to mixed meals. Am J Clin Nutr 1988;47:53–56.
12 Jenkins DJA, Wolever TMS, Jenkins AL: Starchy foods and glycemic index. Diabetes Care 1988; 11:149–159, refs 29–35.
13 Williams SR: Nutrition and Diet Therapy. St Louis, Mosby, 1993, pp 668–669.
14 Williams SR: Nutrition and Diet Therapy. St Louis, Mosby, 1993, p 661.

15 Nestle M: Mediterranean diets: Historical and research overview. Am J Clin Nutr 1995;61(suppl): 1313S–1320S.

16 Grmek MD: Diseases in the Ancient Greek World. Baltimore, Johns Hopkins, 1989, pp 52, 57.

17 Grmek MD: Diseases in the Ancient Greek World. Baltimore, Johns Hopkins, 1989, pp 87ff, esp 91.

18 Friedell E: A Cultural History of Greece: Myth and Reality of the Pre-Christian Soul (in Greek). Athens, Poreia, 1994, p 147.

19 For ages of Alexander's generals, see Oxford Class Dict under their names, or other references on early Hellenistic history.

20 On the Mediterranean diets in general, see Am J Clin Nutr 1995, vol 61, suppl. On gharos in Greek or garum in Latin, see for example, Brothwell D, Brothwell P: Food in Antiquity. London, Thames & Hudson, 1969, pp 159–160.

21 Renaud S, Lorgeril M, Delaye J, Guidolet J, Jacquard F, Mamelle N, Martin J-L, Monjaud I, Salen P, Toubol P: Cretan Mediterranean diet for prevention of coronary heart disease. Am J Clin Nutr 1995;61(suppl):1360S–1367S.

22 Keys A: Coronary heart disease in seven countries. Circulation 1970;41(suppl):1–211.

23 Grmek MD: Diseases in the Ancient Greek World. Baltimore, Johns Hopkins, 1989, pp 80–81.

24 For early contribution to the glycemic index, see Jenkins DJA, Wolever TMS, Taylor RH, Barker H, Fielden H, Baldwin JM, Bowling AG, Newnan HC, Jenkins AL, Goff DY: Glycemic index of foods: A physiological basis for carbohydrate exchange. Am J Clin Nutr 1981;34:362–366. For the latest compilation of the glycemic index of over 500 foods, see Foster-Powell K, Brand Miller J: International tables of glycemic index. Am J Clin Nutr 1995;62(suppl):871S–893S.

25 Foster-Powell K, Brand Miller J: International tables of Glycemic Index. Am J Clin Nutr 1995; 62(suppl):871S–893S, No 428.

26 Foster-Powell K, Brand Miller J: Am J Clin Nutr 1995;62(suppl):871S–893S, sweet potato No 446, 447, 559; taro No 558; yams No 449.

27 Brothwell D, Brothwell P: Food in Antiquity. London, Thames & Hudson, 1969, pp 111–112.

28 Isaiah 39:1.

29 On various aspects of vanadium for living organisms, see Mervyn L 1989: Vitamins and Minerals. London, Thorsons, 1989, under vanadium. Also Davies S, Stewart A: Nutritional Medicine. London, Pan, 1987, p 77. Equally, Brooks RR: Geobotany and Biogeochemistry in Mineral Exploration. New York. Harper & Row, 1972, p 97, table 11.2.

30 Hanfmann GMA: Oxford Class Dict, under Maenads.

31 On the average amount of vanadium in igneous rocks, see Brooks RP: Geobotany and Biogeochemistry in Mineral Exploration. New York, Harper & Row, 1972, p 227. For the vanadium occurrence in bauxites, see Johnstone SJ, Johnstone MG: Minerals for the Chemical and Allied Industries. London, Chapman & Hall, 1961, p 686. For the concentration of vanadium in bauxitic weathering products, see Jones WR: Minerals in Industry. Harmondsworth, Penguin, 1963, p 284.

32 Brooks RP: Geobotany and Biogeochemistry in Mineral Exploration. New York, Harper & Row, 1972, p 27.

33 Athenaeus: Deipnosophists (transl Gulick CB). London, Heinemann, 1960, vol II, 56f, 57a.

34 Unlike today, there were many such animals in Greece outside of Attica at the time; see Flaceliere R: La vie quotidienne en Grece au siècle de Pericles. Paris, 1959, pp 227–228.

35 Mervyn L: Vitamins and Minerals. London, Thorsons, 1989, under vanadium.

36 Novak FA: The Pictorial Encyclopedia of Plants and Flowers. London, Paul Hamlyn, 1966, p 229.

37 The unaltered serpentinites of Lockris, to the NW of Boeotia, contain an average of 29 ppm of vanadium, while the bauxitic laterites derived from them contain an average of 529 ppm. No doubt similar conditions prevail in neighboring Boeotia, as they do in more distant Euboea; see Valeton I, Biermann M, Reche R, Rosenberg F: Genesis of nickel laterites and bauxites in Greece during the Jurassic and Cretaceous and their relation to ultrabasic parent rocks. Ore Geology Reviews 1987;2:359ff, esp 375, table 4, and passim.

Connie Phillipson, PhD, Institute of Paleonutrition Studies,
Box 3771, GR–10210 Athens (Greece)

Simopoulos AP (ed): Nutrition and Fitness: Evolutionary Aspects, Children's Health,
Programs and Policies. World Rev Nutr Diet. Basel, Karger, 1997, vol 81, pp 49–60

....

Evolutionary Aspects of Exercise

Loren Cordain[a], *Robert W. Gotshall*[a], *S. Boyd Eaton*[b]

[a] Department of Exercise and Sport Science, Colorado State University,
Fort Collins, Colo.;
[b] Department of Radiology, Emory University School of Medicine, Atlanta, Ga., USA

As a species, human work (exercise) capacities and limitations are a result of our species-specific anatomical and physiological characteristics, which in turn are defined by our genetic constitution. Similar to all other organisms, the human genome was shaped by environmental selective pressures over eons of evolutionary experience. As hominids evolved and became separate from pongids between 6.3 and 7.7 million years ago (MYA), in response to selective pressures, they developed specific structural and functional characteristics which allowed them to exploit environmental niches which were previously unavailable to their pongid ancestors. Consequently, the selective pressures of the ecological niche which hominids occupied were responsible for shaping those genetic characteristics which are unique to our species (including anatomical and physiological parameters influencing our exercise capacities, limitations and requirements). Examination of both the hominid fossil record and structural and functional differences between modern humans and primates provides insight into the evolutionary changes which occurred in human anatomy and physiology which directly influenced the exercise capacities of contemporary men and women. Further, by studying modern-day hunter-gatherer societies, it is possible to not only develop models of optimal exercise patterns for fitness, but to evaluate how the discordance between the activity patterns of modern sedentary societies and hunter-gatherer societies is implicated in a wide variety of chronic degenerative diseases which plague contemporary man.

Table 1. The main events of human evolution [adapted from ref. 1]

Years ago	Epoch	Development
7,500,000		hominid-pongid divergence
	late Miocene	
4,200,000	Pliocene	bipedal *Australopithecus anamensis* present
3,900,000		*Australopithecus afarensis* present
		Australopithecine divergence
2,000,000		*Homo habilis* present
1,700,000	early Pleistocene	*Homo erectus* present
400,000		archaic *Homo sapiens* appears
230,000		*Homo sapiens neanderthalensis* appears
	late Pleistocene	
45,000		*Homo sapiens sapiens* (anatomically modern) appears
	latest Pleistocene	
10,000		agricultural revolution
	Holocene	
200		industrial revolution

Changes in Hominid Anatomy/Physiology Impacting Exercise Capacities

The evolution of the human species can ultimately be traced to the origin of life itself. However, the distinctive structural and functional features which characterize our species have occurred following the evolutionary split between pongids (apes) and hominids (upright, bipedal primates) 6.3–7.7 MYA (table 1) [1]. Evolutionary changes in hominid anatomy/physiology which have had the greatest impact upon our present day exercise capacities include the development of an upright bipedal gait; increases in cranial capacity and body size associated with changes in dietary quality; the attenuation of body hair and the subsequent development of a highly efficient sweat gland system. In conjunction with these basic anatomical and functional alterations were changes in behavioral complexity which led to increased tool use which in turn is associated with a decreased upper and lower limb robustness [2] (fig. 1).

Bipedalism
The first hominids to walk fully upright (*Australopithecus anamensis*) appear in the fossil record between 3.9 and 4.2 MYA [3] in East Africa coincident with climatic changes in which large areas of the tropical rain forest

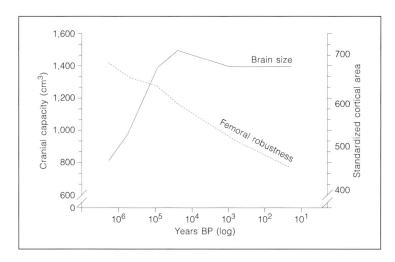

Fig. 1. Changes in percent femoral cortical area [(cortical area/periosteal area) × 100] relative to changes in cranial volume over the course of the evolution of the genus Homo. Adapted from Ruff et al. [2].

were replaced by a more open woodland [4]. *A. anamenis* perhaps represents the ancestral species of the better known Australopithecine, *Australopithecus afarensis* (table 1). *A. afarensis* exhibited sexual dimorphism (weight: 30–70 kg, height 1–1.5 m) and had a cranial capacity of 400–500 ml [5]. *A. afarensis* did not make stone tools and because they maintained a more ape-like body with relatively longer arms and shorter legs than contemporary men, these hominids may have been well adapted to both arboreal and terrestrial environments [6]. Analysis of both fossil footprints and pelvic/leg bone structure indicate that *A. afarensis* walked/ran with a mechanical efficiency similar or superior to modern humans [7].

Although it is not entirely clear which specific environmental pressures were ultimately responsible for the evolution of bipedal locomotion, a number of potential advantages have been identified. An upright, bipedal gait raises the level of the head and provides for a greater visual field for location of food, water and predators in a more open woodland environment [8]. Additionally, bipedalism frees the hands to carry food and other objects during locomotion [7].

More importantly, from an exercise standpoint, bipedalism may be more energy efficient than a comparable quadrupedal posture for standing/walking but not for running. Whereas the oxygen cost of running in man (0.212 ml/g/km) is approximately twice that of other mammals [9], the oxygen cost of human walking is at least as economical as the walking of typical mammalian quadrupeds [10, 11]. Moreover, the difference in energy expenditure for adult humans between their erect and resting (supine) postures is less than that for a quadrupedal animal [12]. Collectively, these data suggest that bipedalism for the most frequent hominid posture (standing/walking) resulted in an energy savings which may have produced a slight but meaningful selective advantage.

Thermoregulation

An upright posture would have had selective advantage for an exercising, diurnal hominid in a hot, sunny woodland or savanna environment because it would reduce the surface area of the body exposed to the sun and thereby reduce the thermal load [13]. Because *A. afarensis* was a biomechanically efficient walker and runner [7] and because their daily range increased substantially with the evolution of bipedalism [14], it has been argued that they may have begun to evolve a more complex eccrine sweat gland system which would have allowed them to run considerable distances under a hot tropical sun without overheating [15]. Further, the evolution of a 'naked' skin (attenuation of body hair size) would have increased the rate at which sweat could be evaporated from the surface of the skin and therefore would have increased the evaporative cooling efficiency of the cutaneous sweat glands [15].

The adaptive value of man's elaborate eccrine system has been largely attributed to its facilitation of heat dissipation during running [16]. The ability to rapidly run considerable distances without overheating would have had obvious survival advantages for bipedal hominids during locomotion in more open woodland and savanna environments. Escape from predators and location and transport of food, infants and other objects would have been facilitated by an efficient evaporative cooling system.

Cranial Capacity and Body Enlargement

The first hominids likely to have made stone tools, *Homo habilis*, had body dimensions similar to *A. afarensis*, but a slightly larger cranial capacity (~750 ml). Increasingly, it has been recognized that in order for a larger, more metabolically active brain to have evolved, an increase in dietary quality (caloric density) had to occur [17–19].

Throughout evolutionary history, carnivorous mammals have always maintained a proportionately larger brain size relative to body size when compared to their herbivorous prey [20]. Because proportionately larger brains are more metabolically active, in order to fuel their increased energetic demands they either require an increase in dietary quality, a reduction in the size and metabolic rate of another tissue, or both [17]. Carnivores have evolved their

Table 2. Metabolic parameters in primates [adapted from ref. 21]

Species	Sex	Weight kg	RMR kcal	TEE kcal	Ratio (TEE/ RMR)	PA-EE kcal	Day range km
Nonhuman primate							
Pan troglodytes	M	39.5	1,036	1,510	1.46	474	4.8
	F	29.8	839	1,144	1.36	305	3.0
Fossil hominids							
Australopithecus afarensis		37.1	1,149	1,824	1.59	675	
Homo habilis		48.0	1,404	2,387	1.70	983	
Homo erectus		53.0	1,517	2,731	1.80	1,214	
Homo sapiens (early)		57.0	1,605	2,889	1.80	1,284	
Modern hunters-gatherers							
Kung	M	46.0	1,275	2,178	1.71	903	14.9
	F	41.0	1,170	1,770	1.51	600	9.1
Ache	M	59.6	1,549	3,327	2.15	1,778	19.2
Acculturated modern humans							
Homo sapiens (office worker)[1]	M	70.0	1,694	2,000	1.18	306	0
	F	55.0	1,448	1,679	1.16	231	0
Homo sapiens (runner)[2]	M	70.0	1,694	2,888	1.70	1,194	12.1

RMR = Resting metabolic rate; TEE = total energy expenditure; PA-EE = energy expenditure attributed to physical activity.
[1] Sedentary office worker [22].
[2] Runner running 12.1 km/h [22].

larger, more metabolically active brains at the expense of a smaller gut. This adaptation can occur because less digestive energy is required to extract food energy from the nutrient dense lipids and proteins in animal foods than from plant foods of low digestibility.

As hominids increasingly included animal foods in their diet, there was a relative increase in brain size and a reduction in their gut size [17] similar to carnivores. These changes were associated with increased behavioral complexity which in turn led to an increased daily range and an increased total energy expenditure (TEE) (table 2). By 1.7 MYA, *H. habilis* was succeeded by *Homo erectus* who stood as tall as contemporary humans [23, 24] and based upon cortical bone thicknesses and diameters [2] was quite heavily muscled and therefore was likely stronger than most modern humans.

Besides being powerfully muscled, *H. erectus* likely had aerobic capacities similar to modern men. Pongids and Australopithecines have rib cages which narrow as they move upward in order to accommodate the extremely powerful muscle groups of the pectoral girdle which are used during arboreal locomotion [17]. Therefore, ventilation of the lungs was probably mainly dependent upon the movements of the diaphragm and would have been less effective than in *H. erectus*, in which the upper part of the rib could have been raised to enlarge the thorax during inspiration [17].

With the appearance of *H. erectus*, hominids not only became taller, but there was a relative decrease in maximal pelvic breadth relative to stature [24]. This relative increase in body linearity would have allowed the (surface area/body mass) ratio to remain favorable for heat dissipation during aerobic activities such as running even though absolute body size had increased from earlier hominids. A relative increase in body linearity may have also facilitated a greater stride length [16] for greater efficiency during running. Regardless of the mechanisms involved, it is clear that the wider rib cages of *H. erectus* and their tall slender physiques facilitated high level aerobic activities in hot climates.

H. erectus (the Kenyan version is sometimes referred to as *H. ergaster*) walked out of Africa by at least 1 MYA or perhaps earlier and colonized eastern Asia but not Europe. Archaic *Homo sapiens* (*Homo heidelbergensis*) inhabited Europe by 400,000–500,000 thousand years ago or perhaps even much earlier [25] and probably represents ancestors of the well-known Neanderthals (*Homo sapiens neanderthalensis*) [26]. Anatomically, modern human beings first appear in the fossil record 90,000–100,000 years ago in the Near East and Africa, and the first truly modern humans, complete with art, culture and sophisticated tools are recognizable 40,000 years ago. Until the agricultural revolution 10,000 years ago, all hominids occupied the hunter-gatherer niche, and regular daily activity utilizing both endurance and strength pathways was essential for all but the most infirm individuals. Consequently, by studying living groups of hunters-gatherers, it is possible to examine the physical activity patterns to which we are genetically adapted so that insight can be gained in determining optimal exercise levels for modern, sedentary societies.

Metabolic Considerations in Primates, Hunters-Gatherers and Contemporary Humans

Activity Patterns in Primates, Hominids and Modern Hunters-Gatherers

Table 2 contrasts the metabolic rates and activity patterns of primates, fossil hominids, modern hunters-gatherers, sedentary office workers and a modern runner. It can be seen that as body weight increases, resting metabolic rate (RMR) increases proportionately. This relationship is well established across mammalian species such that RMR scales to the 3/4th power of body weight [27]. As hominids evolved, they became larger; consequently RMR increased [21]. Additionally, as the tropical forest gave way to more open woodland and savanna environments, caused by prolonged drying periods [4, 28], food resources became less abundant and more dispersed [29]. Therefore, it is probable that early members of the genus *Homo* would have had to increase their daily range [14] and thereby increase the physical activity component (PA-EE) of their total daily energy expenditure (TEE). Since human body size has remained essentially constant since the first appearance of *H. erectus* [24], then the ratio of TEE/RMR in table 2 reflects (ignoring the small thermic effect of food ~5–10% TEE) changes in activity levels which have occurred during the evolution of hominids. The mean estimated (TEE/RMR) ratio (1.87) for hominids since the appearance of full-sized humans *(H. erectus)* represents the activity level for which our species is genetically adapted. The TEE/RMR ratio of sedentary office workers (1.18) denotes activity levels which have previously not been encountered in our species and which are clearly discordant with our genetic requirements.

From table 2, it can be seen that hunter-gatherer males typically spend between 19.6–24.7 kcal/kg/day in physical activity whereas the sedentary office worker would expend only 4.4 kcal/kg/day. Even if a 3.0-mile walk (minimal health benefits suggested by the American College of Sports Medicine [30]) were added to the office workers activities, the resulting value of 8.7 kcal/kg/day would be significantly lower than that which would be normal for our pre-agricultural ancestors. Only when higher level activities are engaged in (say running 12.1 km/h for 60 min) do modern sedentary workers simulate the energy expenditures of our stone age ancestors.

'Primitive' Physical Fitness and Acculturation

Previous studies of modern hunters-gatherers have been compiled by Eaton et al. [31], and mean estimates of maximal oxygen consumption (VO_{2max}) in young men (52 ml/kg/min) would place them in either the excellent to superior fitness classifications as established by Cooper [32] for modern industrialized populations, whereas comparably aged modern men would only have 'fair' fitness levels ($Vo_{2\ max} = 40.8$ ml/kg/min) [31]. Clearly, the normal day-to-day activities of hunters-gatherers, even without the benefit of specific exercises designed to improve cardiorespiratory fitness, produce high levels of endurance.

Rode and Shepherd [33] recently completed a 20-year study (1970–1990) of an Inuit community and were able to document the changes in fitness levels as these hunters-gatherers adopted a more modern, sedentary existence. Not only did activity levels decrease substantially with the adoption of mechanized tools and equipment, but the native diet changed so that it approximated the typical diet of industrialized populations [34]. Associated with these lifestyle changes were increases in body fat, a loss of muscular strength and a decrease in aerobic fitness levels. This native Inuit community is now threatened with 'diseases of civilization' (such as hypertension, cardiovascular disease, and diabetes mellitus) which have been rare until recently [33].

Evolutionary Insights into Exercise, Health and Disease

With the exception of *H. sapiens*, mammals have to work in order to eat: food procurement depends directly upon energy expenditure. Because technological achievement and social organization have disrupted this basic relationship for contemporary humans, low levels of physical exertion have become unprecedentedly common in western, industrialized societies. This departure from exercise patterns which prevailed throughout our evolutionary history has been implicated in the etiology of many chronic degenerative diseases which plague modern-man including diseases of insulin resistance (obesity, non-insulin-dependent diabetes mellitus (NIDDM), hypertension and coronary artery disease) and bone demineralization and fractures.

Diseases of Insulin Resistance
Increasingly it is being recognized that insulin resistance/hyperinsulinemia may be a primary factor in the development of three major diseases (hypertension, NIDDM, coronary artery disease – collectively referred to as 'syndrome X') as well as obesity [35, 36]. These diseases are so epidemic in modern, industrialized societies as to be designated 'diseases of civilizations', since they are rare to nonexistent in less-acculturated societies [31]. The extent to which environmental and genetic factors play in disposing people to these diseases is not clear, however both dietary [37] and exercise [38] patterns seem to play an essential role in the development of syndrome X via their long-term influence upon insulin metabolism.

Acute exercise bouts, either aerobic [39] or strength [40] enhance glucose uptake by skeletal muscle, whereas chronic training is associated with increased skeletal muscle insulin sensitivity and reduced plasma insulin levels [39]. The net effect of an increased insulin sensitivity in conjunction with the increased metabolism of exercise serves to beneficially influence body composition (loss of fat), blood pressure and glucose (lower BP, glucose) and lipid metabolism thereby reducing many of the risk factors for syndrome X.

Relative to activity levels and body composition, trained individuals are similar to our hunter-gatherer ancestors. In response to a glucose load, they secrete less insulin and have lower peak plasma glucose levels than do nonathletes [41]. Twentieth century hunters-gatherers (African San and Efe) and isolated horticulturists (Venezuelan Yanomamo) have insulin sensitivity which is exceptional when compared to that which is considered 'normal' for westernized, affluent individuals [42–44]. When a group of urbanized Australian Aborigines temporarily reverted to a foraging lifestyle, their serum insulin and glucose levels were markedly reduced [45]. For Paleolithic humans, obesity was rare and physical exertion the norm [31]. Accordingly, syndrome X and diseases of hyperinsulinemia would have also been rare.

Bone Demineralization and Fractures

Osteoporosis, a major orthopedic disease (primarily in postmenopausal women), is marked by a decalcification of bone which results in a loss of bone tensile strength that can ultimately lead to fractures. Even though many factors (diet, smoking, genetic and metabolic diseases) including physical activity levels have been suggested as causes of osteoporosis [46], it is likely that the etiology of the disease is multifaceted and no single factor is entirely responsible for its onset [47].

Although there are numerous cross-sectional studies showing that active men and women have a higher bone mineral density (BMD) than those who are sedentary, prospective studies have generally indicated that exercise has a minimal influence upon the postmenopausal decline in BMD [47]. Additionally, studies of BMD using dual-energy X-ray absorptiometers in archaeological skeletons from the Bronze Age [48] and Medieval times [49], during which there was less mechanization and humans presumably were more active, have shown the range of BMD to be similar to modern populations.

Although the most commonly recognized index of bone integrity is BMD, bone structural geometry may be equally, if not more important, in determining a bone's intrinsic strength and ability to resist mechanical stresses [2]. Since BMD is a function of both cortical mass and volume, it is possible to have bones of identical densities but with considerably differing volumes. The greater long bone robustness exhibited by all pre-industrialized humans appears to

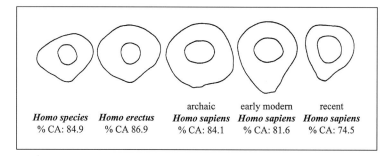

		archaic	early modern	recent
Homo species	*Homo erectus*	*Homo sapiens*	*Homo sapiens*	*Homo sapiens*
% CA: 84.9	% CA 86.9	% CA: 84.1	% CA: 81.6	% CA: 74.5

Fig. 2. Reduction in femoral mid-shaft cross-sectional cortical area from early to recent members of the genus Homo. % CA = [(cortical area/periosteal area) × 100]. Adapted from Ruff et al. [2].

have occurred from relative increases in cortical volume (fig. 2) elicited by greater activity levels [2]. Consequently, the regular loading of skeletal tissue experienced by our pre-industrialized ancestors produced robust, fracture-resistant bones via changes in structural geometry which may have counterbalanced deficiencies in bone mineral content.

Conclusions

Because of the sedentary nature of industrialized societies, exercise is usually viewed as an activity (jogging, walking, swimming, bicycle riding, aerobics, weight lifting, etc.) separate from daily activities, done during leisure time to improve fitness or strength. In contrast, in living hunters-gatherers, exercise results from the daily muscular activity needed to adequately function within the hunter-gatherer niche. Food and water procurement, social interaction, escape from predators, and homeostatic maintenance evoke obligatory movements, and these movements needed to carry out life's functions represent the genetically established exercise patterns of man prior to the agricultural revolution of 10,000 years ago. Although human lifestyles have changed almost inconceivably since the advent of the agricultural revolution and the more recent industrial revolution, our exercise capacities, limitations and requirements remain the same as those selected by natural selection for our stone age ancestors. Deviation from these intrinsic exercise patterns established long ago inevitably results in dysfunction and disease.

References

1 Eaton SB, Konner M: Paleolithic nutrition: A consideration of its nature and current implications. N Engl J Med 1985;312:283–289.

2 Ruff CB, Trinkaus E, Walker A, Larsen CL: Postcranial robusticity in Homo. I. Temporal trends and mechanical interpretation. Am J Phys Anthrop 1993;91:21–53.

3 Leakey MG, Feibel CS, McDougall I, Walker A: New four-million-year-old hominid species from Kanapoi and Allia Bay, Kenya. Nature 1995;376:565–571.

4 Behrensmeyer AK, Cooke HS: Paleoenvironments, stratigraphy, and taphonomy in the African Pliocene and early Pleistocene; in Delson E (ed): Ancestors: The Hard Evidence. New York, Liss, 1985, pp 60–62.

5 Wood BA: Evolution of australopithecines; in Jones S, Martin R, Pilbeam D (eds): The Cambridge Encyclopedia of Human Evolution. Cambridge, Cambridge University Press, 1992, pp 231–240.

6 Stern JT, Susman RL: The locomotor anatomy of Australopithecus afarensis. Am J Phys Antrop 1983;60:279–317.

7 Lovejoy CO: Evolution of human walking. Sci Am 1988;259:118–125.

8 Shipman P: Scavenging or hunting in early hominids: Theoretical framework and tests. Am Anthrop 1986;88:27–43.

9 Taylor CR, Heglund NC, Maloiy GO: Energetics and mechanics of terrestrial locomotion. Part 1. J Exp Biol 1982;97:1–21.

10 Rodman PS, McHenry HM: Bioenergetics and the origin of hominid bipedalism. Am J Phys Anthrop 1980;52:103–106.

11 Tucker VA: The cost of moving about. Am Sci 1975;63:413–419.

12 Arbitol MM: Effect of posture and locomotion on energy expenditure. Am J Phys Anthrop 1988; 77:191–199.

13 Wheeler PE: The influence of bipedalism on the energy and water budgets of early hominids. J Hum Evol 1991;21:117–136.

14 Foley R: Early man and the red queen: Tropical African community evolution and hominid adaptation; in Foley R (ed): Hominid Evolution and Community Ecology. New York, Academic Press, 1984, pp 85–110.

15 Wheeler PE: The influence of the loss of functional body hair on the water budgets of early hominids. J Hum Evol 1992;23:379–388.

16 Carrier DR: The energetic paradox of human running and hominid evolution. Curr Anthrop 1984; 25:483–495.

17 Aiello LC, Wheeler PE: The expensive tissue hypothesis. Curr Anthrop 1995;36:199–221.

18 Leonard WR, Robertson ML: Evolutionary perspectives on human nutrition: The influence of brain and body size on diet and metabolism. Am J Hum Biol 1994;6:77–88.

19 Milton K: Diet and primate evolution. Sci Am 1993;269:86–93.

20 Jerison HJ: The Evolution of the Brain and Intelligence. New York, Academic Press, 1973, pp 287–319.

21 Leonard WR, Robertson ML: Nutritional requirements and human evolution: A bioenergetics model. Am J Hum Biol 1992;6:77–88.

22 Heyward VH: Advanced Fitness Assessments and Exercise Prescription. Champaign, Human Kinetics Publishers, 1991, pp 326–331.

23 Brown F, Harris J, Leakey R, Walker A: Early homo erectus skeleton from west lake Turkana, Kenya. Nature 1985;316:788–792.

24 Ruff CB: Climate and body shape in hominid evolution. J Hum Evol 1991;21:81–105.

25 Carbonell E, Bermudez de Castro JM, Arsuaga JL, Diez JC, Rosas A, Cuenca-Bescos G, Sala R, Mosquera M, Rodriguez XP: Lower pleistocene hominids and artifacts from Atapuerca-TD6. Science 1995;269:826–830.

26 Tattersall I: The Last Neanderthal. New York, Macmillan, 1995, pp 38–73.

27 Klieber M: The Fire of Life. New York, Wiley, 1961, pp 212.

28 deMenocal PB: Plio-Pleistocene African climate. Science 1995;270:53–59.

29   Foley R, Lee PC: Finite social space, evolutionary pathways, and reconstructing hominid behavior. Science 1989;243:901–906.

30   Kenney WL (ed): American College of Sports Medicine: ACSM's Guidelines for Exercise Testing and Prescription. Baltimore, Williams & Wilkins, 1995, pp 153–167.

31   Eaton SB, Konner M, Shostak M: Stone agers in the fast lane: Chronic degenerative diseases in evolutionary perspective. Am J Med 1988;84:739–749.

32   Cooper KH: The Aerobics Way. New York, Bantam Books, 1977, pp 257–266.

33   Rode A, Shephard RJ: Physiological consequences of acculturation: A 20-year study of fitness in an Inuit community. Eur J Appl Physiol 1994;69:516–524.

34   Rode A, Shephard RJ: Prediction of body fat content in an Inuit community. Am J Hum Biol 1994; 6:249–254.

35   Reaven GM: Role of insulin resistance in human disease. Diabetes 1988;37:1595–1607.

36   Reaven GM: Role of insulin resistance in human disease (syndrome X): An expanded definition. Ann Rev Med 1993;44:121–131.

37   Simopoulos AP: Is insulin resistance influenced by dietary linoleic acid and trans fatty acids? Free Rad Biol Med 1994;17:367–372.

38   Horton ES: Exercise and decreased risk of NIDDM. N Engl J Med 1991;325:196–198.

39   Horton ES: Exercise and physical training: Effects on insulin sensitivity and glucose metabolism. Diabetes Metab Rev 1986;2:1–17.

40   Fluckey JD, Hickey MS, Brambrink JK, Hart KK, Alexander K, Craig BW: Effects of resistance exercise on glucose control in normal and glucose-intolerant subjects. J Appl Physiol 1994;77: 1087–1092.

41   Kriska AM, Blair SN, Pereira MA: The potential role of physical activity in the prevention of non-insulin dependent diabetes mellitus: The epidemiological evidence. Exerc Sports Sci Rev 1994;22: 121–143.

42   Joffe BI, Jackson WU, Thomas ME, Toyer MG, Keller P, Pimstone BL: Metabolic responses to oral glucose in the Kalahari Bushman. Br Med J 1971;4:206–208.

43   Merimee TJ, Rimoin DL, Cavalli-Sforza LL: Metabolic studies in the African Pygmy. J Clin Invest 1972;51:395–401.

44   Spielman RS, Fajans SS, Neel JV, Pek S, Floyd SC, Oliver WJ: Glucose tolerance in two unaccultur-ated Indian tribes of Brazil. Diabetologia 1982;23:90–93.

45   O'Dea K: Marked improvement in carbohydrate and lipid metabolism in diabetic Australian Abori-gines after temporary reversion to traditional lifestyle. Diabetes 1984;33:596–603.

46   Geelhoed EA, Criddle A, Prince RL: The epidemiology of osteoporotic fracture and its causative factors. Clin Biochem Rev 1994;15:173–178.

47   Drinkwater BL: 1994 C.H. McCloy research lecture: Does physical activity play a role in preventing osteoporosis? Res Quart Exerc Sport 1994;65:197–206.

48   Kneissel M, Boyde A, Hahn M, Teschler-Nicola M, Kalchhauser G, Plenk H: Age- and sex-dependent cancellous bone changes in a 4000y BP population. Bone 1994;15:539–545.

49   Ekenman I, Eriksson AV, Lindgren JU: Bone density in Medieval skeletons. Calcif Tissue Int 1995; 56:355–358.

Loren Cordain, PhD, Department of Exercise and Sport Science, Colorado State University, Fort Collins, CO 80523 (USA)

Simopoulos AP (ed): Nutrition and Fitness: Evolutionary Aspects, Children's Health,
Programs and Policies. World Rev Nutr Diet. Basel, Karger, 1997, vol 81, pp 61–71

....

Genetic Variation: Nutrients, Physical Activity and Gene Expression

Artemis P. Simopoulos

Center for Genetics, Nutrition and Health, Washington, D.C., USA

The interaction between genetic and environmental factors influences human development and is the foundation for health and disease. Genetic factors determine susceptibility to disease and environmental factors determine which genetically susceptible individuals will be affected. Nutrition and physical activity (exercise) are two of the most important environmental factors in maintaining health and well-being. Hippocrates in defining the concept of positive health stated the importance of man's constitution (what today we call genetics) and said that if there is a deficiency in food or exercise the body will fall sick.

Major advances have occurred over the past 15 years in the fields of both genetics and nutrition [1–7]. Using the tools of molecular biology and genetics, research is defining the mechanisms by which genes influence nutrient absorption, metabolism and excretion, taste perception, and degree of satiation; and the mechanisms by which nutrients influence gene expression. Furthermore, advances in molecular and recombinant deoxyribonucleic acid (DNA) technology have led to exquisite studies in the field of genetics and the recognition in a much more specific way, through DNA sequencing, how unique each one of us is, and the extent to which genetic variation occurs in human beings. The importance of the effects of genetic variation has been extensively studied and applied by pharmacologists in drug development and evaluation of drug metabolism and adverse reactions to drugs [8–12]. The landscape of preventive medicine is changing and in the past two decades physicians, geneticists, nutritionists, and exercise physiologists began to study the effects of genetic variation, gene-nutrient interactions and the effects of exercise in the management of chronic diseases [1–3, 13–18].

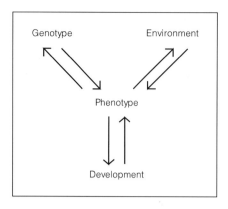

Fig. 1. Relationships among genes, environment, and development are dynamic.

Genetic Individuality and Polymorphisms

Each human being in being unique, is exceptional in some way. Individuality is determined by *genes* (both major genes and modifiers), *constitutional factors* (age, sex, developmental stage, parental factors) and *environmental factors* (time, geography, climate, socioeconomic status, occupation, education and diet). All sorts of interactions among these three sources of variation are possible.

Genes do not provide an unalterable blueprint but merely a set of options, each more or less conditional, and to be taken up according to what is being experienced as well as what has been experienced. Thus, gene-environment interaction must be described in the context of development and in a dynamic, dialectical mode [19, 20] (fig. 1).

Common alleles (variants at a single locus) or polymorphisms form the basis of human diversity, including the ability to handle environmental challenge. How extensively variable the human species is depends on the methods used for its determination. At the DNA level there is a great deal of variation whereas at the level of protein diversity there is much less. In humans and practically all organisms examined, 30% of loci have polymorphic variants (defined as two or more alleles with frequency of at least 1% or more) in the population. An average individual is heterozygous at about 10% of the loci. Alleles that confer selective advantage in the heterozygous state are likely to have increased in prevalence because of positive selection acting on variants. Changes in nutritional environment will affect heritability of the variant phenotypes that are dependent, to a lesser or greater degree, on the nutrient environment for their expression [21].

In the past decade methodologic advances in molecular genetics have facilitated the study of inherited diseases at the DNA level. Specific gene segments from genomic DNA or cDNA can be selectively amplified through the polymerase chain reaction (PCR) and subsequently analyzed by various techniques to detect mutations or polymorphisms. Polymerase chain reaction has revolutionized DNA analysis and it is beginning to have a substantial effect in clinical medicine. In vitro amplification of DNA has facilitated the approach to genetic diseases at the DNA level.

Role of Nutrients and Exercise in Gene Expression

Nutrients influence gene expression either through the mediation of hormones or directly. Over the past 10 years there has been an increase in the use of concepts evolved from molecular biology in the study of food components and essential nutrients, as well as exercise, as factors in the control of gene expression [5].

Nutrients Influence Gene Expression

In terms of chronic diseases, particularly relevant are the effects of dietary cholesterol and fatty acids on gene expression. Dietary cholesterol exerts a profound inhibitory effect on the transcription of the gene for HMG-CoA reductase responsible for cholesterol synthesis [22]. Dietary polyunsaturated fatty acids (PUFA) suppress the hepatic mRNA production of fatty acid synthase for lipoproteinemia in adult and weanling rats. This ability to suppress the abundance of mRNAs for lipogenic proteins is dependent on the degree of fatty acid unsaturation. Eicosapentaenoic acid (EPA) and docosahexaenoic acid (DHA) in the form of fish oils are thus more effective than arachidonic acid (AA) [23]. Dietary n–3 fatty acids reduce levels of mRNA for platelet-derived growth factor (PDGF) [24] and for IL-1β indicating regulation at the transcriptional level [25] (table 1). These effects of n–3 fatty acids may explain their beneficial effects in decreasing mortality in patients with one episode of myocardial infarction [26] and in decreasing the severity of disease in patients with arthritis, psoriasis, and ulcerative colitis [27].

Exercise Influences Gene Expression

The effects of exercise on lipoprotein lipase (LPL) expression in different tissues and the mechanisms involved are now being elucidated. Studies in normal volunteers by Seip et al. [28] indicate that in skeletal muscle, exercise training increased the mean LPL mRNA level by 117%, LPL protein mass by 53% and total LPL enzyme activity by 35%, whereas no changes occurred

Table 1. Effects of polyunsaturated fatty acids on several genes encoding enzyme proteins involved in lipogenesis, growth factors, and inflammation

Fatty acid	Lipogenesis [23] FAS, S14 SCDI, SCDII ACC, ME	Growth factors [24] PDGF mRNA	Inflammation [25] IL-1β mRNA
LA	↓		
LNA	↓		
AA	↓	↑	↑
EPA	↓	↓	↓
DHA	↓↓	↓	↓

↓ = Suppress or decrease; ↑ = induce or increase.

in adipose tissue. It appears that the exercise stimulus is specific for skeletal muscle. Exercise decreased serum triglycerides, total cholesterol and very-low-density lipoprotein (VLDL) while it increased high-density lipoprotein (HDL) [28]. In this study as in previous studies changes in muscle but not adipose tissue heparin-releasable LPL activity were inversely correlated with changes in triglycerides [29]. Muscle is probably the major site of triglyceride removal in humans, and increased LPL enzyme activity may be a major factor in the generation of HDL. This increase in LPL activity appears to be at the level of transcriptional, or pretranslational mechanisms leading to the improvement in circulating lipids seen with physical activity.

The larger intracellular pool of active LPL enzyme induced by exercise in the study of Seip et al. [28], would readily replenish LPL at the capillary endothelium and ultimately result in enhanced triglyceride lipolysis. Increased LPL expression in muscle would provide a source of fatty acids for oxidation and may protect against fatigue, allowing the performance of more work and perhaps an improved sense of well-being.

Seip et al. [28] concluded: 'The major finding of our study is that exercise regulation of muscle LPL expression in humans can be pretranslational. This raises fundamental physiological questions about the time course of the LPL message response after exercise and the intensity of exercise required to elicit this response. We speculate that more vigorous skeletal muscle contraction will result in proportionally more LPL expression, suggesting that for the induction of muscle LPL gene expression, as with most things in life, harder work will be associated with greater benefits.'

Studies in dogs indicate that chronic exercise increases the production of endothelium-derived relaxing factor (EDRF/nitric oxide, NO), thus contributing to the beneficial effects of exercise on the cardiovascular system. A potential mechanism that may contribute to the increased production of nitrite in vessels may be the induction of endothelial cell NO synthase (ECNOS). Sessa et al. [30] showed that steady-state mRNA levels of ECNOS were significantly higher in exercised dogs. In rat studies Apple et al. [31] showed that gene expression of creatine kinase isoenzymes appear to be partially controlled at the level of transcription following exercise training.

Some exercise adaptations induce the differential expression of genes that encode components of the contractile apparatus, metabolic pathways, organelle systems and membrane components. Transgenic animals are useful in determining the molecular basis for the activation of enzymes during prolonged submaximal exercise [32].

Physical exercise is characterized by an increase in lean body mass and by healthy changes in serum lipid levels and carbohydrate metabolism. There is a decrease in adipose tissue, an increase in high-density lipoprotein concentration, a decrease in cholesterol level, and lower blood pressure. Changes in carbohydrate metabolism include an increase in glucose uptake and an increase in insulin sensitivity in muscle; mobilization of free fatty acids from the adipose tissue; and a higher capacity to oxidize free fatty acids in the muscle cell. Exercise produces a metabolic status that maintains energy balance. Thus, the interrelationships of nutrition and physical activity are evident.

Genetic Variation and Dietary Response

Dietary recommendations have been developed by governments and associations for the control of coronary artery disease [33]. The guidelines recommend a decrease in dietary saturated fat and cholesterol intake. Drugs have been developed and used to lower plasma cholesterol levels. Yet it has been known for at least 20 years that the response of plasma cholesterol concentration to cholesterol feeding is heterogeneous although the mechanisms only recently are being understood [34–37]. Some examples of the advances in our understanding of the mechanisms involved follow.

Apo E Variants
In certain situations the response to diet appears to be determined by the genetic variant of apolipoprotein as, for example, in the case with Apo E variants. Three common isoforms are present in the population and are designated by their isoelectric focusing positions: Apo E2, Apo E3, and Apo E4.

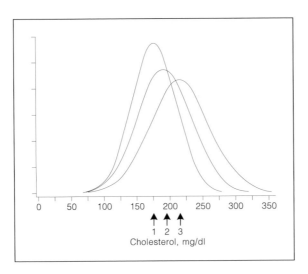

Fig. 2. Cholesterol distribution for selected male populations: 1 = mean for Japan; 2 = mean for Minnesota; 3 = mean for Finland. From Sing et al. [39].

This polymorphism results in six common phenotypes: three homozygous (E2/2, E3/3, and E4/4) and three heterozygous (E4/2, E4/3, and E3/2). The Apo E3/3 phenotype is the most common, occurring in approximately 60% of the population. Therefore, Apo E3 is considered the parent form of this protein, and Apo E2 and Apo E4 are its variants [38].

Genetic variation within a population contributes to differences in average plasma cholesterol levels (fig. 2) [39]. In every population studied thus far, the E4 allele is associated with an increase and the E2 allele is associated with a decrease in plasma cholesterol levels [40]. The relative frequency of the E3 allele is less than 0.79 in every Caucasian (high cholesterol) sample and exceeds 0.84 for Chinese and Japanese (low cholesterol) samples. The E4, but not the E2, allele is significantly increased in the Finnish population which has the highest levels of plasma cholesterol and risk of coronary artery disease among the populations studied [41]. The Japanese have a lower frequency of Apo E4/4, lower serum cholesterol levels and a lower death rate of coronary heart disease (table 2) [39].

On a low-fat/high-cholesterol diet individuals with Apo E4/4 phenotype respond with an increase in serum cholesterol whereas those with Apo E2/2, 3/2, 3/4 do not show an increase. On a low-fat/low-cholesterol diet all variants show a decrease in serum cholesterol. Thus, serum cholesterol response to dietary cholesterol is phenotype dependent [42]. The interaction between lipo-

Table 2. A comparison of CHD mortality rates, plasma cholesterol levels, percent saturated fat in the diet and relative frequencies of Apo E allelles in Japan, Minnesota and Finland

CHD Mortality	Japan	Minnesota	Finland
	600	1,400	2,100[a]
	130	350	700[b]
Mean plasma cholesterol, mg/dl	178.26	190.70	217.00
Percent saturated fat in diet	2.90	16.20	23.70
Apo E2	0.04	0.08	0.04
Apo E3	0.85	0.78	0.73
Apo E4	0.11	0.14	0.23

[a] Males (age 65–74); per 100,000.
[b] Females (age 45–64); per 100,000.
Modified from Sing et al. [39].

protein responsiveness to dietary manipulation and Apo E phenotype has been the subject of several investigations [43]. A recent meta analysis study supports the concept that Apo E4 allele is associated with an increased LDL cholesterol response to dietary manipulation [44]. On a low-fat/low-cholesterol diet the magnitude of LDL cholesterol lowering is twice as great in males as in females. The lowering of LDL cholesterol in Apo E3/4 males was (23%) which was significantly greater than that observed in Apo E3/3 (14%) or Apo E3/2 (13%), suggesting that males with the Apo E3/4 are more responsive to diets restricted in saturated fat and cholesterol than Apo E3/3 males [44].

Whereas Apo E4 is associated with hypercholesterolemia the variant forms of Apo E2 are associated with the development of type III hyperlipoproteine-mia and the accumulation of chylomicron and VLDL remnants in the plasma [38]. Only 1 person in 50 with Apo E2 variants develops hypertriglyceridemia. Since triglyceride removal is genetically determined, increases in either energy intake, trans fatty acid intake, or carbohydrate intake (particularly in women), all of which stimulate triglyceride synthesis, lead to hypertriglyceridemia. Besides diet, obesity, diabetes and hypothyroidism facilitate Apo E2 variant gene expression [38].

Additional studies show that women of the Apo E3/2 phenotype stand to benefit the least from a high polyunsaturate:saturate (P:S) diet because of reduction in the more 'protective' high-density lipoprotein cholesterol (HDL-C), whereas men of the Apo E4/3 phenotype showed the greatest improvement in the LDL/HDL ratio. Therefore, a general recommendation to increase the polyunsaturated content of the diet in order to decrease plasma cholesterol level and the risk for coronary artery disease is not appropriate for women with Apo 3/2 phenotype [45].

Oat bran has been shown to decrease serum cholesterol levels in some studies but not in others. Recently, it was shown that only subjects with Apo E3/3 phenotype had a hypocholesterolemic response to oat bran at 4 weeks but no change was noted in individuals with Apo E4/4 or 4/3 type [46]. Thus, specific genetic information is needed to define the optimal diet for an individual. General recommendations usually lead to inconclusive studies or show lack of benefit.

Apo A-IV-2 Variant

The variant apolipoprotein (Apo) allele Apo A-IV-2 decreases the response of the plasma cholesterol concentration to dietary cholesterol [47]. In the US about 1 in 7 in the population is heterozygote and carries the Apo A-IV-2 allele. The homozygote state is Apo IV-1/1. Increasing dietary cholesterol from 200 to 1,100 mg/day by the addition of four eggs/day, total cholesterol increased 22 mg/dl in the Apo IV-1/1 group and only 6 mg/dl in the Apo IV-1/2 group. The mean plasma low-density-lipoprotein (LDL) cholesterol increased by 19 in the Apo IV-1/1 group and only 1 mg/dl in the Apo A IV-1/2 group. Neither group had any changes in the plasma triglycerides or HDL cholesterol concentration. These results again show the genetic effects of the response to dietary cholesterol.

LDL Subclass Patterns

Gradient gel electrophoresis analyses of LDL have been used to classify subjects into two groups based on distinct LDL subclass patterns, denoted A and B. LDL subclass phenotypes are also associated with different lipoprotein responses to reduced fat diets. About 25% of the population carries a common heritable lipoprotein phenotype characterized by a predominance of small dense LDL particles (pheno B) which is associated with higher triglycerides and lower HDL levels, and increased risk of coronary artery disease. This pheno B is found after age 20 in males and after menopause in females [48–50]. Pheno A refers to a large buoyant LDL. The effect of a high- and low-fat diet on subjects with the two different LDL subclasses was investigated by Dreon and Krauss [51]. A low-fat diet (24% of energy) led to a reduction of pheno B but some of the pheno A individuals changed to pheno B on the low-fat diet. A low-fat/high-carbohydrate diet confers no benefit to pheno A but is beneficial to pheno B. Low-fat diets are in fact detrimental to pheno A individuals. Such findings indicate the need to know the specific phenotype before specific dietary recommendations are made.

Studies on the effects of exercise consistently show small increases in LDL size. Long distance runners have a decrease in mass of smaller denser LDL particles determined by ultracentrifugation [52]. In a 1-year study of diet-induced and exercise-induced weight loss in sedentary, moderately overweight men, the size of the major LDL subclass increased 2.4 A (p<0.05) in the exercise group compared to the control group [53]. Neither of these studies examined LDL subclass phenotypes and it is unlikely that the small, 2–3 A changes would result in changes in phenotypes.

Conclusions

Genetic variation influences the response to diet. Physical activity influences gene expression. Proper diet and exercise have similar beneficial effects. Because of differences in gene frequency, dietary habits and activity levels, universal dietary recommendations are inappropriate. Instead, knowledge of specific genes and response to exercise should guide dietary advice for health, and in the prevention and management of chronic diseases.

References

1   Simopoulos AP, Childs B (eds): Genetic variation and nutrition. World Rev Nutr Diet. Basel, Karger, 1990, vol 63, pp 1–300.
2   Simopoulos AP, Herbert V, Jacobson B: Genetic Nutrition: Designing a Diet Based on Your Family Medical History. New York, Macmillan, 1993.
3   Goldbourt U, de Faire U, Berg K: Genetic Factors in Coronary Heart Disease. Dordrecht, Kluwer Academic Publishers, 1994.
4   Velazquez A, Bourges H (eds): Genetic Factors in Nutrition. Orlando, Academic Press, 1984.
5   Rucker R, Tinker D: The role of nutrition in gene expression: A fertile field for the application of molecular biology. J Nutr 1986;116:177–189.
6   Castro CE, Towle HC: Nutrient-genome interaction. Fed Proc 1986;45:2392–2393.
7   Berdanier CD, Hargrove JL (eds): Nutrition and Gene Expression. Boca Raton, CRC Press, 1993.
8   Gonzalez FJ, Skoda RC, Kimura S, Umeno M, Zanger UM, Nebert DW, Gelboin HV, Hardwick JP, Meyer UA: Characterization of the common genetic defect in humans deficient in debrisoquine metabolism. Nature 1988;331:442–446.
9   Price-Evans DA: In Kalow W, Goedde HW, Agarwal DP (eds): Ethnic Differences in Reactions to Drugs and Xenobiotics. New York, Liss, 1986, pp 491–526.
10   Price-Evans DA, Harmer D, Downham DY, Whibley EJ, Idle JR, Ritchie J, Smith RL: The genetic control of sparteine and debrisoquine in metabolism in man with new methods of analyzing biomodal distributions. J Med Genet 1983;20:321–329.
11   Idle JR: Poor metabolizers of debrisoquine reveal their true colours. Lancet 1989;ii:1097.
12   Wolf CR, Moss JE, Miles JS, Gough AC, Spurr NK: Detection of debrisoquine hydroxylation phenotypes. Lancet 1990;336:1452–1453.
13   Wood PD, Stefanick ML, Dreon DM, Frey-Hewitt B, Garay SC, Williams PT, Superko HR, Fortmann SP, Albers JJ, Vranizan KM: Changes in plasma lipids and lipoproteins in overweight men during weight loss through dieting as compared with exercise. N Engl J Med 1988;319: 1173–1179.

14   Vena JE, Graham S, Zielezny M, Brasure J, Swanson MK: Occupational exercise and risk of cancer. Am J Clin Nutr 1987;45(suppl):318–327.

15   Simopoulos AP: Nutrition and fitness. JAMA 1989;261:2862–1863.

16   Pariza MW, Simopoulos AP (eds): Proceedings of the Conference on Calories and Energy Expenditure in Carcinogenesis. Am J Clin Nutr 1987;45(suppl):149–372.

17   Simopoulos AP, Pavlou KN (eds): Nutrition and Fitness for Athletes. Part I. Proceedings of the Second International Conference on Nutrition and Fitness, Athens, 1992. World Rev Nutr Diet. Basel, Karger, 1993, vol 71.

18   Simopoulos AP (ed): Nutrition and Fitness in Health and Disease. Part II. Proceedings of the Second International Conference on Nutrition and Fitness, Athens, 1992. World Rev Nutr Diet. Basel, Karger, 1993, vol 72.

19   Childs B: Genetic variation and nutrition. Am J Clin Nutr 1988;48:1500–1504.

20   Lewontin RC: Gene, organism and environment; in Bendall DS (ed): Evolution from Molecules to Man. Cambridge, Cambridge University Press, 1983.

21   Scriver CR: Nutrient-gene interactions: The gene is not the disease and vice versa. Am J Clin Nutr 1988;48:1505–1509.

22   Osborn TF, Goldstein JL, Brown MS: 5′-End of HMG-CoA reductase gene contains sequences responsible for cholesterol-mediated inhibition of transcription. Cell 1985;42:203–212.

23   Clarke SD, Jump DB: Regulation of hepatic gene expression by dietary fats: A unique role for polyunsaturated fatty acids; in Berdanier CD, Hargrove JL (eds): Nutrition and Gene Expression. Boca Raton, CRC Press, 1993.

24   Kaminski WE, Jendraschek C, Kiefl R, von Schacky C: Dietary ω–3 fatty acids lower levels of PDGF mRNA in human mononuclear cells. Blood 1993;81:1871–1875.

25   Urakaze M, Sugiyama E, Xu L, Auron P, Yeh E, Robinson D: Dietary marine lipids suppress IL-1B mRNA levels in lipopolysaccharide stimulated monocytes (abstract). Clin Res 1991:23.

26   Burr ML, Fehily AM, Gilbert JF, Rogers S, Holliday RM, Sweetnam RM, Elwood PC, Deadman NM: Effect of changes in fat, fish and fibre intakes on death and myocardial reinfarction: Diet and reinfarction trial (DART). Lancet 1989;ii:757–761.

27   Simopoulos AP: Omega–3 fatty acids in health and disease and in growth and development. Am J Clin Nutr 1991;54:438–463.

28   Seip RL, Angelopoulos TJ, Semenkoveich CF: Exercise induces human lipoprotein lipase gene expression in skeletal muscle but not adipose tissue. Am J Physiol 1995;268:E229–E236.

29   Nikkila EA: Role of lipoprotein lipase in metabolic adaptation to exercise and training; in Borensztajn J (ed): Lipoprotein Lipase. Chicago, Evener, 1987, pp 187–199.

30   Sessa WC, Pritchard K, Seyedi N, Wang J, Hintze TH: Chronic exercise in dogs increases coronary vascular nitric oxide production and endothelial cell nitric oxide synthase gene expression. Circ Res 1994;74:349–353.

31   Apple FA, Billadello JJ: Expression of creatine kinase M and B mRNAs in treadmill trained rat skeletal muscle. Life Sci 1994;55:585–592.

32   Tsika RW: Transgenic animal models. Exerc Sport Sci Rev 1994;22:361–388.

33   Truswell AS: Evolution of dietary recommendations, goals, and guidelines. Am J Clin Nutr 1987; 45:1060–1072.

34   Beynen AC, Katan MB, Van Zutphen LFM: Hypo- and hyperresponders: Individual differences in the response of serum cholesterol concentration to changes in diet. Adv Lipid Res 1987;22:115–171.

35   Miettinen TA, Kensaniemi YA: Cholesterol absorption: Regulation of cholesterol synthesis and elimination and within-population variations of serum cholesterol levels. Am J Clin Nutr 1989;49: 629–635.

36   Nestel PJ, Poyser A: Changes in cholesterol synthesis and excretion when cholesterol intake is increased. Metabolism 1976;25:1591–1599.

37   Glatz JF, Turner PR, Katan MD, Stalenhoef AF, Lewis B: Hypo- and hyperresponse of serum cholesterol level and low density lipoprotein production and degradation to dietary cholesterol in man. Ann NY Acad Sci 1993;676:163–179.

38   Mahley RW, Weisgraber KH, Innerarity TL, Rall SC: Genetic defects in lipoprotein metabolism: Elevation of atherogenic lipoproteins caused by impaired catabolism. JAMA 1991;265:78–83.

39   Sing CF, Kaprio J, Perusse L, Moll PP: Genetic differences in risk of disease within and between populations; in Simopoulos AP, Childs B (eds): Genetic Variation and Nutrition. World Rev Nutr Diet. Basel, Karger, 1990, vol 63, pp 220–235.

40   Davignon J, Gregg RR, Sing CF: Apo E polymorphism and atherosclerosis. Arteriosclerosis 1988; 8:1–21.

41   World Health Organisation MONICA Project: Myocardial infarction and coronary deaths in the World Health Organisation MONICA project: Registration procedures, event rates and case fatality in 38 populations from 21 countries in four continents. Circulation 1994;90:583–612.

42   Miettinen TA, Gylling H, Vanhanen H: Serum cholesterol response to dietary cholesterol and apolipoprotein E phenotype. Lancet 1988;ii:1261.

43   Dallongeville J: Apolipoprotein E polymorphism and atherosclerotic risk; in Goldbourt U, de Faire U, Berg K (eds): Genetic Factors in Coronary Heart Disease. Dordrecht, Kluwer, 1994, pp 289–298.

44   Lopez-Miranda J, Ordovas JM, Mata P, Lichtenstein AH, Clevidence B, Judd JT, Schaefer EJ: Effect of apolipoprotein E phenotype on diet-induced lowering of plasma low density lipoprotein cholesterol. J Lipid Res 1994;35:1965–1975.

45   Cobb MM, Teitlebaum H, Risch N, Jekel J, Ostfeld A: Influence of dietary fat, apolipoprotein E phenotype, and sex on plasma lipoprotein levels. Circulation 1992;86:849–857.

46   Uusitupa MIJ, Ruuskanen E, Makinen E, Laitinen J, Toskala E, Kervinen K, Kesaniemi YA: A controlled study on the effect of beta-glucan-rich oat bran on serum lipids in hypercholesterolemic subjects: Relation to apolipoprotein E phenotype. J Am Coll Nutr 1992;11:651–659.

47   McCombs RJ, Marcadis DE, Ellis J, Weinberg RB: Attenuated hypercholesterolemic response to a high-cholesterol diet in subjects heterozygous for the apolipoprotein A-IV-2 allele. N Engl J Med 1994;331:706–710.

48   Austin MA, King M-C, Vranizan KM, Newman B, Krauss RM: Inheritance of low-density lipoprotein subclass patterns: Results of complex segregation analysis. Am J Hum Genet 1988;43:838–846.

49   Austin MA, Breslow JL, Hennekens CH, Buring JE, Willett WC, Krauss RM: Low-density lipoprotein subclass patterns and risk of myocardial infarction. JAMA 1988;260:1917–1921.

50   Krauss RM: Low-density lipoprotein subclasses and risk of coronary artery disease. Curr Opin Lipidol 1991;2:248–252.

51   Dreon DM, Krauss RM: Low density lipoprotein subclass phenotypes are associated with differing lipoprotein responses to reduced-fat diets (abstract). Circulation 1991;84(suppl II);681.

52   Williams PT, Krauss RM, Wood PD, Lindgren FT, Giotas C, Vranizan KM: Lipoprotein subfractions of runners and sedentary men. Metabolism 1986;35:45–52.

53   Williams PT, Krauss RM, Vranizan KM, Labers JJ, Terry RB, Wood PDS: Effects of exercise-induced weight loss on low density lipoprotein subfraction in healthy men. Arteriosclerosis 1989; 9:623–632.

Artemis P. Simopoulos, MD, The Center for Genetics, Nutrition and Health,
2001 S Street, NW, Suite 530, Washington, DC 20009 (USA)

Simopoulos AP (ed): Nutrition and Fitness: Evolutionary Aspects, Children's Health,
Programs and Policies. World Rev Nutr Diet. Basel, Karger, 1997, vol 81, pp 72–83

....

Genetics, Response to Exercise, and Risk Factors: The HERITAGE Family Study[1]

Jack H. Wilmore[a], *Arthur S. Leon*[b], *D.C. Rao*[c], *James S. Skinner*[d],
Jacques Gagnon[e], *Claude Bouchard*[e]

[a] Department of Kinesiology and Health Education, The University of Texas at
Austin, Tex.;
[b] School of Kinesiology and Leisure Studies, University of Minnesota, Minneapolis,
Minn.;
[c] Division of Biostatistics and Departments of Genetics and Psychiatry, Washington
University Medical School, St. Louis, Mo., and
[d] Department of Kinesiology, Indiana University, Bloomington, Ind., USA;
[e] Physical Activity Sciences Laboratory, Laval University, Québec, Canada

It is commonly recognized that a physically active lifestyle is associated
with a decreased risk for a variety of morbid conditions. The conclusion of
a recent International Consensus Conference on the relationship between
physical activity, fitness and health was that there is ample evidence from
experimental studies, as well as cross-sectional and prospective data from
large-scale epidemiological studies, that regular exercise improves health-
related fitness and has important positive effects on general wellness, morbidity and mortality [1]. However, the consensus document specified that additional studies were needed to improve our understanding of the contribution
of inherited factors in determining changes in risk profiles in response to
lifestyle modifications, such as those seen when individuals engage in regular
exercise. From the population viewpoint, regular exercise can potentially
reduce the risk associated with the incidence of coronary artery disease,
hypertension, type II diabetes mellitus, osteoporosis, obesity and other degenerative conditions [1]. Alterations in risk profile brought about by regular
exercise are thought to be mediated by favorable effects on such factors

[1] Adapted, in part, from Bouchard et al.: The HERITAGE Family Study: Aims, design,
and measurement protocol. Med Sci Sports Exerc 1995;27:721–729, with permission.

as plasma lipids and lipoproteins, insulin sensitivity, body fat content and distribution, particularly upper body fat and abdominal visceral fat, blood pressure, steroid and glucocorticoid hormonal profile, cardiac output, stroke volume and oxygen transport capacity.

Since cardiovascular disease and noninsulin dependent diabetes account for over half of the deaths and a large fraction of the health care costs in the US, there is considerable interest in understanding the role of regular exercise on risk factors related to these diseases, as well as the individual variation in the response to regular exercise. A large body of research clearly indicates that maximal oxygen uptake ($\dot{V}O_{2\,max}$), cardiac output, and the metabolic pathways related to tissue substrate availability are all biological characteristics that can favorably adapt to exercise training [2–4]. For instance, $\dot{V}O_{2\,max}$ typically increases by about 20–30% after several months of training [3, 5]. The activity of key enzymes of skeletal muscle oxidative potential often increases by 50% and, at times, doubles pretraining values [6–9].

While few experiments have been designed to document the importance of variation in the response to regular exercise, those which looked for these individual differences have found them [10–12]. For instance, in one experiment, Lortie et al. [5] trained 24 sedentary young adults for 20 weeks. The cycle ergometer training program was the same for each subject and fully monitored. While the average $\dot{V}O_{2\,max}$ rose 0.6 liters/min or 26%, gains ranged from 7 to 87%. Large individual differences in sensitivity to regular exercise have also been reported for endurance performance [5, 13], cardiorespiratory adaptation to exercise [14] and changes in skeletal muscle enzyme activities [9, 13, 15], plasma lipoproteins and apoproteins [16, 17], adipose tissue metabolism [18, 19], and insulin response to a glucose load [20]. Individual differences in response to training for these biological characteristics typically range from a low of 0% to a high of about 50–100% of the pre-exercise values.

What factors contribute to such variation in response to regular exercise? Briefly, age and gender, as well as prior exercise experience, did not seem to contribute significantly to individual differences in trainability in 18- to 30-year-old subjects. The major causes of variation in endurance training response included the pretraining level of the phenotype and undetermined genetic characteristics, as reported in several separate experiments conducted with sets of identical twins [12]. These experiments suggest that there are high-, low-, and no-responder genotypes in the response of $\dot{V}O_{2\,max}$ to regular exercise. Although this phenomenon has been documented primarily in young adults of both sexes, it is probably also present in middle-aged and older individuals, as well as for most of the cardiovascular disease and diabetes risk factors. Moreover, the problem has been investigated only with identical twins [12]. The need for a more detailed study of the phenomenon in parents and their offspring was thus apparent. Thus, the HERITAGE Family Study (HEalth, RIsk factors, exercise Training And GEnetics) has been designed to document the role of the genotype in the cardiovascular, metabolic and hormonal responses to aerobic exercise-training. A consortium of 5 universities in the US and Canada are involved in carrying out the study.

Aims of the HERITAGE Family Study

The overall objective of the HERITAGE project is to study the role of the genotype in cardiovascular, metabolic and hormonal responses to aerobic exercise training and the contribution of regular exercise to changes in several cardiovascular disease and diabetes risk factors. It addresses the following major aims:

(a) To extend our understanding of the genetic epidemiology of the following selected risk factors, with emphasis on changes observed with regular exercise: blood lipids, lipoproteins, apoproteins and lipolytic enzymes; glucose tolerance and insulin sensitivity; systolic and diastolic blood pressure at rest and during exercise; body weight, total body fat, regional fat distribution, and abdominal visceral fat; and steroid and glucocorticoid hormone levels. The issues to be resolved will be related to the heritability of each phenotype and its response to exercise training, the contribution of a specific paternal or maternal effect, sex-limited effects, major gene effects and related segregation patterns.

(b) To extend our understanding of the genetic epidemiology of aerobic exercise tolerance, its functional determinants and their response to training. Major dependent variables include $\dot{V}O_{2 \, max}$, cardiac output, stroke volume, and adaptation to submaximal exercise and training. This will allow the determination of potential mechanisms responsible for the large variation in physiological response to a standardized endurance exercise training program.

(c) To investigate a number of physiological and epidemiological issues independent of potential familial aggregation such as: the role of regular exercise on various risk factors; differences between genders, between young and middle-age adults, and between Caucasians and African-American subjects; and effects of other lifestyle components, particularly smoking, nutrient intake, alcohol intake, sleep habits, on various phenotypes.

(d) Our ultimate objective is to perform association and linkage studies between risk factor and performance phenotypes, especially as they relate to responses to exercise training, with a panel of candidate genes and other genetic markers.

Design and Sampling

The study design calls for the recruitment of 90 two-generational nuclear families of Caucasian descent and 40 families of African-American ancestry, each with both biological parents and at least three biological children. However, due to the sociodemographic characteristics of African-American families, they often tend to be uniparental (mostly the mother and her children from multiple marriages), and tend not to have many children in the required age range who are full sibs. Therefore, some African-American families will involve fewer than 5 subjects. We expect that about half of the African-American families will each have five or more members. The sample is expected to comprise a total of about 650 individuals. Families will be selected such that all participating members are within 17–65 years of age (age of children: 17–40; age of parents: 65 and less), 'sedentary' for 3 months prior to beginning the study and essentially in good health. The participating individuals will be studied before and again after a 20-week standardized training program, providing the opportunity to assess the familiality of response to regular exercise. A control group of families is not included in the design for several reasons: previous studies have documented appreciable changes in both fitness and risk factor variables; the pretraining measures provide approximate control levels; and the enormous cost associated with obtaining data on control families.

Measurement Protocol

The study was approved by each participating institution's review board for including human subjects in research. Written informed consent is obtained from each study participant. Each subject receives USD 1,000 in incremental payments for successful completion of the study, i.e. after completing the 20-week training program plus the pre- and posttraining battery of tests.

Health screening includes a health history, physical examination, a resting electrocardiogram (ECG) and an exercise test with ECG monitoring. Subjects also complete at baseline a health habit questionnaire, including smoking and alcohol consumption habits; The ARIC-Baecke Physical Activity Questionnaire [21, 22]; The Willett Food Frequency Questionnaire to assess usual food nutrient patterns [23]; The Minnesota Eating Pattern Assessment Tool (EPAT) to evaluate dietary fat sources [24, 25]; a menstrual history; and a detailed family history questionnaire. The health habit and EPAT questionnaires are repeated at the midpoint of training (week 10), at which time participants are counseled again not to change baseline health habits. They are administered again at the end of training.

Anthropometric measurements taken before and after training include standing height, body weight and a series of 8 skinfold measurements using Harpenden calipers [26]. Circumferences of the upper arm, waist and hip (buttocks) are also obtained [27]. Underwater weighing is performed in the postabsorptive state before and after training to determine body density, fat mass, fat-free mass and relative body fat [28]. A correction is made for residual lung volume by the oxygen dilution principle [29, 30]. Abdominal visceral fat and abdominal subcutaneous fat is quantified before and after training by the method of Sjöström et al. [31]. This technique involves computed axial tomography (CT scan) at the level of the disk between lumbar vertebrae 4 and 5 using the same protocol at all centers and the scans are sent to Laval University for review.

Resting blood pressure measurements are made twice prior to the start of exercise training and at 24 and 72 h posttraining. Subjects are tested before 11:00 a.m. in the postabsorptive state with no caffeine-containing beverages and tobacco products for at least 2 h prior to measurements. Measurements are performed in a quiet room at neutral ambient temperature (24–25 °C) with the lights dimmed and subjects rested for at least 5 min in a reclining chair with legs elevated and the chair's back support reclined at about 45° from the ground. Blood pressure is determined using a properly fitted cuff connected to a Colin STBP-780 automated unit. Ear phones are worn by the technicians during measurements to confirm blood pressure values.

Three exercise tests are administered both prior to and at the conclusion of the training period. All tests are conducted on a stationary cycle ergometer (Ergo-Metrics 800S from Sensormedics) in the sitting position. The first test is to establish the participant's $\dot{V}O_{2\,max}$, as well as the normality of the exercise electrocardiogram in the pretraining test. During the second test of each battery, participants exercise at 50 W and at 60% of their $\dot{V}O_{2\,max}$ determined in the initial test for about 8 min at each power output to determine steady-state $\dot{V}E$, F_EO_2, F_ECO_2, RER, systolic and diastolic blood pressure, heart rate, cardiac output, and stroke volume. During the third and final test of each battery, the participant repeats the 50 W and power output at 60% of $\dot{V}O_{2\,max}$ of the second test, after which the power output is increased to 80% $\dot{V}O_{2\,max}$ for 3 min, and then continues to increase until the subject reaches exhaustion. The same variables are monitored during the second and third tests. In addition, a venous catheter is inserted in the left arm to obtain blood samples at rest, during exercise at 50 W, 60 and 80% $\dot{V}O_{2\,max}$, and immediately upon completion of the maximal test. Blood samples are analyzed for glucose, free fatty acids, lactate and total proteins. Metabolic measurements and cardiac output (CO_2 rebreathing technique) are determined using a SensorMedics 2900 metabolic cart, blood pressure with a Colin STBP-780 automated blood pressure monitor, and heart rate from the electrocardiogram. The same test battery is administered post-training.

To measure plasma lipid and lipoprotein levels, blood samples are collected from an antecubital vein into vacutainer tubes containing EDTA. Samples are taken in the morning after a 12-hour fast while the subjects are in a supine position. Cholesterol (C) and triglycerides (TG) levels are determined in plasma and in lipoprotein fractions by enzymatic methods using the Technicon RA-1000 analyzer. Plasma VLDL (d < 1.006 g/ml) are isolated by ultracentrifugation [32] and the HDL fraction obtained after precipitation of LDL in the infranatant (d > 1.006 g/ml) with heparin and $MnCl_2$ [33]. The C and TG content of the infranatant fraction are measured before and after the precipitation step. Apo B concentration is measured in plasma and the infranatant (LDL-Apo B) by the rocket immunoelectrophoretic method of Laurell [34]. Apo A-1 concentration is also measured in the infranatant fraction. The concentrations of LDL-C, LDL-TG and VLDL-Apo B are obtained by difference. The cholesterol content of HDL_2 and HDL_3 subfractions prepared by the precipitation method [35] is also determined. Apo E phenotype is measured by an isoelectrofocusing method. LPL and H-TGL activities are measured in plasma obtained from 12-hour-fasted subjects, 10 min after i.v. injection of heparin (60 IU/kg body weight). Enzyme activities are measured by a modification of the method of Nilsson-Ehle and Ekman [36].

An intravenous glucose tolerance test is performed in the morning after an overnight fast. Blood samples are collected through a venous catheter from an antecubital vein for a total of 16 time points over 3 h to determine plasma glucose, insulin and connecting peptide (C-peptide) concentrations. Plasma glucose is enzymatically measured [37], whereas plasma insulin is measured by radioimmunoassay with polyethylene glycol separation [38]. C-peptide is measured by a modification of the method of Heding [39] using polyethylene glycol precipitation [38]. A colorimetric micromethod [40] is used to measure free fatty acids.

After extraction, measurements of serum steroid levels are performed by specific radioimmunoassays [41]. The following steroids are assayed: androstenedione, testosterone, dihydrotestosterone, androsterone glucuronide, androstane-3a,17β-diol glucuronide, pregnenolone fatty acid esters and dehydroepiandrosterone and its fatty acid. Progesterone, 17-hydroxyprogesterone, cortisol, aldosterone, estradiol, and dehydroepiandrosterone sulfate are determined using Diagnostic Product Corporation kits. Sex hormone binding globulin is also determined using a commercial kit.

Permanent lymphoblastoid cell lines are established for each individual of the cohort to insure a continuous source of DNA. Given the wealth of performance, physiological, metabolic and health data that will be gathered, such an approach is of the utmost importance. Lymphoblastoid cell lines are obtained by transformation of human lymphocytes with the Epstein-Barr virus (EBV). Such cell lines grow well in culture, have an infinite life span and present a chromosomal stability over the years [42]. The procedure requires the isolation of monocyte cells, the transformation with the EBV and the cryopreservation of the transformed cell lines. Cell lines are also thawed occasionally to check cell viability.

The Training Program

Each family member is trained on a cycle ergometer, 3 times a week, for 20 weeks using the same standardized training protocol in each of the 4 Clinical Centers. Training intensity is adjusted for individual differences in $\dot{V}O_{2\,max}$. The intensity and/or duration of the training program is adjusted each 2 weeks, such that the subjects are working at the heart rate associated with 75% $\dot{V}O_{2\,max}$ for 50 min during the last 6 weeks; this allows an adequate total energy turnover for a sufficient time period, increasing the chances to induce changes in many of the variables under investigation. The power output of the cycle ergometer is adjusted automatically by computer to the heart rate response of the subject at all times during all training sessions, and the computer stores both mean heart rate and mean power output for each minute of each training session. All training sessions are supervised on site.

Data Entry and Management

A distributed data entry system has been developed for HERITAGE using SAS as a data management tool. The system was developed by the Data Coordinating Center in St. Louis. Each Clinical Center enters the data on its own PC and sends it to the Data Coordinating Center on diskette, where it is collated into a master database. As errors are discovered, reports are generated back to the Clinical Centers, where the errors are resolved and the revised data resent to the Data Coordinating Center.

Data Analysis Plan

The data analysis plan presented here provides an overview of the types of data analyses that are planned. Racial differences will be investigated by analyzing data on African-American families and on Caucasian families separately whenever possible and necessary. We remain alert to the possibility of modifying these plans as other pertinent information becomes available, such as from analysis of partial data. In addition to using the traditional epidemiological model of response to exercise training, the following analyses will be conducted.

Path Analysis

We propose to analyze the familial aggregation of many variables using the methods of path analysis, which enables a resolution of genetic, familial environmental, and random environmental effects [43]. This is accomplished by defining the covariance among relatives, and in the case of the multivariate analysis, the covariance among phenotypes both within individuals and among relatives, in terms of parameters of a model of genetic and environmental effects. For many of the pretraining variables in the performance domain, the familial aggregation of which is not well known, univariate analyses of one variable at a time will provide that information. Although these analyses will be interesting contributions in their own right, they will be equally useful in guiding additional analyses using complex multivariate models. Using multivariate models [44, 45], it is possible to test whether the same genetic influences are acting on multiple measures. For example, the question of whether genetic influences on a cardiovascular risk variable in sedentary individuals (pretraining) are identical to the influences on the variable in trained individuals can be modeled and explicitly tested. Similarly, it is possible to assess in detail relationships between the mechanism underlying the change in a variable in response to exercise training and its baseline level. Finally, some of these models will also enable investigations of temporal trends in family resemblance [46].

Segregation Analysis

Segregation analysis will be carried out to investigate possible major gene effects on a variety of phenotypes such as, for example, change in a certain risk factor [47–49]. Underlying genetic models assume that the phenotype results from the joint and independent effects of an autosomal locus and residual multifactorial effects. Segregation at the major locus is modeled using general transmission probabilities that are the probabilities of the genotypes AA, Aa, and aa transmitting the A allele; Mendelian transmission holds when these probabilities are 1, 1/2, and 0, respectively. Test of the major gene hypothesis involves contrasting the model in which the major gene parameters are set to zero against the general model in which those parameters are estimated. For those variables exhibiting evidence of a major gene effect, tests on transmission probabilities will be performed to protect against an incorrect inference in the presence of environmentally-induced major effects. More recent models also permit combined path and segregation analysis [50, 51].

For variables that exhibit significant changes in response to exercise training, complex segregation analysis of the change between the pre- and posttraining values will be carried out. The primary purpose of these analyses is to investigate the nature of familial effects, if any, on the observed changes, with special reference to additional major gene effects. This is expected to suggest whether specific genotypes are associated with the ability to respond to exercise training. A dichotomy of 'responders' and 'nonresponders', defined in terms of whether there is a marked change between the pre- and posttraining values, may be useful. For some of the more informative variables, analyzing the segregation of the 'responder' status in families may provide important information.

Association and Linkage Studies

Associations between dichotomized response variables and a host of genetic markers will be tested. This approach serves two purposes. There is a possibility of identifying alleles associated with a higher/lower mean response in polygenically (multifactorially) determined variables. In addition, a preliminary notion of potential linkage relationships can be ascertained for those variables influenced by major genes.

If evidence of a single gene affecting the change in any variable after exercise training is found, then an attempt to implicate a particular gene will be made via linkage analysis with likely candidate-gene markers. Candidate genes can be identified on the basis of biological considerations, or in light of the associations revealed in the preliminary screening. Linkage analyses will be carried out using standard computer programs such as LINKAGE and LIPED. Lod scores, which denote measures of the relative odds that two loci are linked at particular recombination fractions versus unlinked, will be calculated.

Conclusions

The HERITAGE family study will document the role of the genotype in the cardiovascular, metabolic and hormonal responses to aerobic exercise-training. A consortium of 5 universities in the USA and Canada are involved in carrying out the study. A total of 90 Caucasian families and 40 African-American families with both parents and three or more biological adult offspring are being recruited, tested, exercise-trained in the laboratory with the same program for 20 weeks, and retested. $\dot{V}O_2$, RER, blood pressure, heart rate, cardiac output, blood lactate, glucose, and free fatty acids are measured during exercise and $\dot{V}O_{2\,max}$ is determined before and after training. Plasma lipids, lipoproteins and apoproteins, glucose and insulin response to an intravenous glucose load, plasma sex steroids and glucocorticoids, and body fat and fat distribution are assessed. Dietary and activity habits, and other lifestyle components are assessed by questionnaires, prior to, during and after training. A variety of genetic analyses will be undertaken, including heritability studies and major gene effects, for each phenotype and its response to regular exercise. Cell lines are established and DNA sequence variation at a variety of molecular markers will be determined for association and linkage studies.

Acknowledgments

The HERITAGE study is supported by the National Heart, Lung and Blood Institute through the following grants: HL45670 (C. Bouchard, PI), HL47323 (A.S. Leon, PI), HL47317 (D.C. Rao, PI), HL47327 (J.S. Skinner, PI) and HL47321 (J.H. Wilmore, PI).

Thanks are expressed to all the co-principal investigators, investigators, co-investigators, local project coordinators, research assistants, laboratory technicians, and secretaries who are contributing to the study. Finally, the entire HERITAGE consortium is very thankful to those hard-working participating families whose involvement alone demonstrates the feasibility of this study.

References

1   Bouchard C, Shephard RJ, Stephen T (eds): Physical Activity, Fitness, and Health: Consensus Statement. Champaign, Human Kinetics Publishers, 1993, 102 pp.
2   Holloszy JO: Biochemical adaptations in muscle: Effects of exercise on mitochondrial oxygen uptake and respiratory enzyme activity in skeletal muscle. J Biol Chem 1967;242:2278–2282.
3   Pollock ML: The quantification of endurance training programs. Exerc Sport Sci Rev 1973;1: 155–188.
4   Saltin B, Blomqvist G, Mitchell JH, Johnson RL, Wildenthal K, Chapman CB: Response to exercise after bed rest and after training. Circulation 1968;38:1–68.
5   Lortie G, Simoneau JA, Hamel P, Boulay MR, Landry F, Bouchard C: Responses of maximal aerobic power and capacity to aerobic training. Int J Sports Med 1984;5:232–236.
6   Holloszy JO, Coyle EF: Adaptation of skeletal muscle to endurance exercise and their metabolic consequences. J Appl Physiol 1984;56:831–838.
7   Howald H: Training-induced morphological and functional changes in skeletal muscle. Int J Sports Med 1982;3:1–12.
8   Saltin B, Gollnick P: Skeletal muscle adaptability: Significance for metabolism and performance; in Peachy LD, Adrian RH, Geiger SR (eds): Skeletal Muscle. Handbook of Physiology. Maryland, American Physiological Society, 1983, pp 555–631.
9   Simoneau JA, Lortie G, Boulay MR, Marcotte M, Thibault MC, Bouchard C: Effects of two high-intensity intermittent training programs interspaced by detraining on human skeletal muscle and performance. Eur J Appl Physiol 1987;56:516–521.

10   Bouchard C: Genetics of aerobic power and capacity; in Malina RM, Bouchard C (eds): Sport and Human Genetics. Champaign, Human Kinetics, 1986, pp 59–88.

11   Bouchard C, Boulay MR, Simoneau JA, Lortie G, Pérusse L: Heredity and trainability of aerobic and anaerobic performances: An update. Sports Med 1988;5:69–73.

12   Bouchard C, Dionne FT, Simoneau JA, Boulay MR: Genetics of aerobic and anaerobic performances. Exerc Sport Sci Rev 1992;10:27–58.

13   Hamel P, Simoneau JA, Lortie G, Boulay MR, Bouchard C: Heredity and muscle adaptation to endurance training. Med Sci Sports Exerc 1986;18:690–696.

14   Prud'homme D, Bouchard C, Leblanc C, Landry F, Fontaine E: Sensitivity of maximal aerobic power to training is genotype dependent. Med Sci Sports Exerc 1984;16:489–493.

15   Simoneau JA, Lortie G, Boulay MR, Marcotte M, Thibault MC, Bouchard C: Inheritance of human skeletal muscle and anaerobic capacity adaptation to high-intensity intermittent training. Int J Sports Med 1986;7:167–171.

16   Després JP, Bouchard C, Savard R, Tremblay A, Allard C: Lack of relationship between changes in adiposity and plasma lipids following endurance training. Atherosclerosis 1985;54:135–143.

17   Després JP, Moorjani S, Tremblay A, Poehlman ET, Lupien PJ, Nadeau A, Bouchard C: Heredity and changes in plasma lipids and lipoproteins after short-term exercise training in men. Arteriosclerosis 1988;8:402–409.

18   Després JP, Bouchard C, Savard R, Prud'homme D, Bukowiecki L, Theriault G: Adaptive changes to training in adipose tissue lipolysis are genotype dependent. Int J Obes 1984;8:87–95.

19   Savard R, Després JP, Marcotte M, Bouchard C: Endurance training and glucose conversion into triglycerides in human fat cells. J Appl Physiol 1985;58:230–235.

20   Tremblay A, Poehlman ET, Nadeau A, Pérusse L, Bouchard C: Is the response of plasma glucose and insulin to short-term exercise-training genetically determined? Horm Metabol Res 1987;19:65–67.

21   Baecke JAH, Burema J, Frijters JER: A short questionnaire for the measurement of habitual physical activity in epidemiological studies. Am J Nutr 1982;36:936–942.

22   Jacobs DR Jr, Ainsworth BE, Hartman TJ, Leon AS: A simultaneous evaluation of 10 commonly used physical activity questionnaires. Med Sci Sports Exerc 1992;25:81–91.

23   Willett WC, Sampson L, Stampfer MJ, Rosner B, Bain C, Witschi J, Hennekens CH, Speizer FE : Reproducibility and validity of a semi-quantitative food frequency questionnaire. Am J Epidemiol 1985;122:51–65.

24   Hunninghake DB, Mullis RM, Brekke ML, Peters JR, Quiter ES: A simple tool for the assessment of dietary fat intake in clinical populations. Circulation Abstr 60th Sci Sess 1987;76(suppl. IV):35.

25   Peters JR, Brekke MJ, Quiter ES, Mullis RM, Brekke ML, Hunninghake DB: Eating pattern assessment tool: A simple instrument for assessing dietary fat. J Am Diet Assoc 1994;94:1008–1013.

26   Harrison GG, Buskirk ER, Carter JEL, Johnston FE, Lohman TG, Pollock ML, Roche AF, Wilmore J: Skinfold thicknesses and measurement technique; in Lohman TG, Roche AF, Martorell R (eds): Anthropometric Standardization Reference Manual. Champaign, Human Kinetics Books, 1988, pp. 55–80.

27   Callaway CW, Chumlea WC, Bouchard C, Himes JH, Lohman TG, Martin AD, Mitchell CD, Mueller WH, Roche AF, Seefeldt VD: Circumferences; in Lohman TG, Roche AF, Martorell R (eds): Anthropometric Standardization Reference Manual. Champaign, Human Kinetics Books, 1988, pp 39–54.

28   Behnke AR, Wilmore JH: Evaluation and Regulation of Body Build and Composition. Englewood Cliffs, Prentice-Hall, 1974, pp 21–27.

29   Wilmore JH: A simplified method for determination of residual lung volume. J Appl Physiol 1969;27:96–100.

30   Wilmore JH, Vodak PA, Parr RB, Girandola RM, Billing JE: Further simplification of a method for determining residual lung volume. Med Sci Sports 1980;12:216–218.

31   Sjöström L, Kvist H, Cerberblad A, Tylen U: Determination of the total adipose tissue volume in women by computed tomography. Comparison with 40K and tritium techniques. Am J Physiol 1986;250:736–745.

32   Havel RJ, Eder H, Bragdow HF: The distribution and chemical composition of ultracentrifugally separated lipoproteins in human serum. J Clin Invest 1955;34:1345–1353.

33   Burstein M, Samaille J: Sur un dosage rapide du cholestérol lié a- et aux -lipoprotéines du sérum. J Clin Chim Acta 1960;5:609–610.

34   Laurell CB: Quantitative estimation of proteins by electrophoresis in agarose gel containing antibodies. Anal Biochem 1966;15:45–52.

35   Gidez LI, Miller GJ, Burstein M, Slage S, Eder HH: Separation and quantitation of subclasses of human plasma high density lipoproteins by a simple precipitation procedure. J Lipid Res 1982;23: 1206–1233.

36   Nilsson-Ehle P, Ekman R: Specific assays for lipoprotein lipase activities of post-heparin plasma; in Peeters H (ed): Protides of Biological Fluids. Oxford, Pergamon Press, 1978, pp 243–246.

37   Richterich R, Dauwalder H: Zur Bestimmung der Plasmaglukose-Konzentration mit der Hexokinase-Glucose-6-Phosphat-Dehydrogenase Methode. Schweiz Med Wochenschr 1971;101:615–618.

38   Desbuquois B, Aurbach GD: Use of polyethylene glycol to separate free and antibody-bound peptide hormones in radioimmunoassays. J Clin Endocrinol Metab 1971:37:732–738.

39   Heding LG: Radioimmunological determination of human C-peptide in serum. Diabetologia 1975; 11:541–548.

40   Noma A, Okabe H, Kita M: A new colorimetric micro-determination of free fatty acids in serum. Clin Chim Acta 1973;43:317–320.

41   Bélanger A, Caron S, Picard D: Simultaneous radioimmunoassay of progestins, androgens and estrogens in rat testis. J Steroid Biochem 1980;13:185–190.

42   Nilsson K: Establishment of permanent human lymphoblastoid cell lines in vitro; in Bloom BR, David JR (eds): In Vitro Methods in Cell-Mediated and Tumor Immunity. New York, Academic Press, 1976, pp 713–735.

43   Rao DC: Application of path analysis in human genetics; in Krishnaish PR (ed): Multivariate Analysis. Part VI. Amsterdam, North-Holland, 1985, pp 467–484.

44   Hanis CL, Sing CF, Clarke WR, Schrott HT: Multivariate models for human genetic analysis: Aggregation, and tracking of systolic blood pressure and weight. Am J Hum Genet 1983;36: 1196–1210.

45   Vogler GP, Rao DC, Laskarzewski PM, Glueck CJ, Russell JM: Multivariate analysis of lipoprotein cholesterol fractions. Am J Epidemiol 1987;125:706–719.

46   Province MA, Rao DC: A new model for the resolution of cultural and biological inheritance in the presence of temporal trends: Application to systolic blood pressure. Genet Epidemiol 1985;2: 363–374.

47   Bonney GE: On the statistical determination of major gene mechanisms in continuous human traits: Regressive models. Am J Med Genet 1984;18:731–749.

48   Borecki IB, Lathrop GM, Bonney GR, Yaouanq J, Rao DC: Combined segregation and linkage analysis of genetic hemochromatosis using affection status, serum iron, and HLA. Am J Hum Genet 1990;47:542–550.

49   Lalouel JM, Rao DC, Morton NE, Elston RC: A unified model for complex segregation analysis. Am J Hum Genet 1983;35:816–826.

50   Li Z, Bonney GE, Lathrop GM, Rao DC: Genetic analysis combining path analysis with regressive models: The TAU model of multifactorial transmission. Hum Hered 1994;44:305–311.

51   Province MA, Rao DC: General purpose model and a computer program for combined segregation and path analysis (SEGPATH): automatically creating computer programs from symbolic language model specifications. Genetic Epidemiology 1995;12:203–219.

Jack H. Wilmore, PhD, Department of Kinesiology and Health Education, Bellmont Hall 222, The University of Texas at Austin, Austin, TX 78712 (USA)

Simopoulos AP (ed): Nutrition and Fitness: Evolutionary Aspects, Children's Health,
Programs and Policies. World Rev Nutr Diet. Basel, Karger, 1997, vol 81, pp 84–89

....

Summary of Part 2

Gilman D. Grave

National Institute of Child Health and Human Development,
National Institutes of Health, Bethesda, Md., USA

Grave opened the session, cochaired by Maria Hassipidou, by noting that Socrates trod this very ground nearly 2,500 years ago. According to Xenophon's *Memorabilia* Socrates noted at a dinner party while watching a dancing girl perform that he, too, danced every morning in order to lose weight. Others at Xenophon's party attested to Socrates' morning dancing, and one of them had imitated Socrates himself. It is intriguing to remind ourselves at this conference on nutrition and fitness that the Ancient Greeks were aware of the close connection between exercise, weight maintenance, and health. It is also noteworthy that they made long daily peregrinations from home to shrine to agora, pedion (drama), and gymnasium all of which contributed to their fitness, health and longevity. Walter Agard [The Greek Mind, New York, Van Nostrand, 1957, p. 12] has noted that the ancient Greeks attained a high level of civilization without being comfortable (by today's standards).

Stallings discussed the nutritional needs of the excercising child. She noted that few data exist on this subject; however, the nutritional needs of the growing child are paramount and must never be compromised. The extra demands for energy and other nutrients that are superimposed on those of the growing child must be met by additional intake. There is no evidence that pre-exercise loading with carbohydrate (carbo-loading) is helpful or desirable. Nutrient supplements, clearly, are not desirable because they may pave the way for the belief that pills lead to improved health. Any excess nutritional burden posed by strenuous exercise should be met by eating increased quantities of a balanced diet.

If the added nutritional needs imposed by strenuous exercise in prepubertal children are not provided, then postpubertal stunting may ensue owing to nutrient deprivation during the growth spurt followed by epiphyseal union during Tanner Stage V puberty. Stallings also stressed the need for adequate hydration during strenuous exercise. This is especially important for parents and coaches to remember because the sensation of thirst may be under-developed in children.

Stallings also warned against the development of eating disorders in some children who exercise strenuously not for reasons of physical fitness, but rather to keep from gaining weight. These children often have a distorted body image. They are at risk for postpubertal stunting as well as for low calcium intake and poor bone deposition during adolescence. Even nonexercising children and children without eating disorders run the risk of impaired bone deposition, especially girls. Data from NHANES II indicate that girls are consuming < 800 mg calcium/day, despite an RDA of 1,200 mg. Children, especially girls, need to attain as high a peak bone density as possible prior to the onset of their third decade. The greater a girl's peak bone density at age 20, the less likely will she experience osteoporosis later in life. The recent availability of DEXA should help pediatricians get accurate data on their patients' bone mass.

Other than increasing calcium intake in exercising children, there is no known requirement for micronutrient supplementation. No need has ever been shown for additional micronutrients in exercising children.

Even though the data are spotty on determining the additional energy intake needed by exercising children, use of the WHO equation to predict resting energy expenditure (REE) from age, sex, and weight is recommended. Stallings reminded everyone involved in pediatric care to be sensitized to incipient behavior that may lead to either overfeeding and obesity or to anorexia nervosa or anorexia bulimia.

Finally, Stallings stressed the need to form lifelong habits of good nutritional eating and exercising. More research is needed on diet composition and health outcome, as well as specific research on some children who exercise strenuously.

Oja followed. He addressed the paradigm set forth by Blair in Blair, et al. [Exercise and fitness in childhood: Implications for a lifetime of health; in Gisolfi CV, Lamb DR (eds): Perspectives in Exercise and Sports Medicine, vol 2. Youth, Exercise, and Sport. Indianapolis, Benchmark Press, 1989, pp 401–430].

Thesis 1: Childhood exercise ↔ Children's health
Thesis 2: Childhood exercise ↔ Adult health
Thesis 3: Childhood exercise ↔ Adult exercise
Thesis 4: Adult exercise ↔ Adult health

Oja noted that this paradigm raises three possibilities, none of which has been proved definitively: (1) Exercise might directly improve the health of children. This thesis is particularly difficult to prove, since children are generally healthy and active and rarely develop chronic disease in childhood. However, the roots of several chronic diseases begin in childhood, e.g. obesity, hypertension, atherosclerosis. Therefore, proxy measures of risk of these disorders offer the only means of establishing the validity of direction. (2) Even though parameters such as Body Mass Index (BMI), blood pressure, and serum lipids track with various degrees of fidelity from childhood into adulthood there is no good prospective evidence that altering these risk factors by exercise in childhood affects adult outcome favorably in regard to either these proxy measures or to morbidity and mortality.

Similarly, there are no data that support thesis 1, since the real threats to children's health are accidents, cancer, infectious disease, allergies, and congenital malformations. From the standpoint of the general pediatric population exercise in childhood provides no indication of improved health in childhood.

Thesis 4 has support in the literature. There is much evidence that adult exercise benefits adult health, especially if performed for ≥ 30 min most days of the week.

Thesis 3 may be valid. We hope that by enjoying exercise in childhood, children will incorporate exercise into their lifestyle which may track into adulthood. Unfortunately, there is no study that supports this tracking of salutary behavior into adulthood.

Oja continued by noting that active children do have better risk profiles. He also noted that obesity is the most common pediatric disorder. Obesity in childhood can be reversed on a short-term basis by programs of diet and exercise. It has been shown that multifocal interventions engender better and longer-lasting results. Oja noted also that active children have lower blood pressures than sedentary children. However, no prospective study results of this difference are available.

In regard to bone mass, Oja presented data on female tennis players. The bone mineral density of the playing arm in all cases was greater than the nonplaying arm. The differences were much greater in those players who began their tennis career prior to menarche. This study strongly supports the salutary effect of exercise on bone mineral density and bone mass in growing children.

Oja then quoted the recent work of Riddoch and Boreham [1995] who reviewed the literature on self-reported activity assessment. Because these studies all involve self-reporting, there may be a built-in bias towards overestimation of activity. The mean figures derived from the articles ranged from 30 to 80 min/day. Riddoch and Boreham concluded that 60–70% of children are sufficiently active. Oja then reviewed data generated by the National Child and Youth Family Surveys I and II, which examined children in grades 5–12 and grades 1–4, respectively. These studies concluded that 59% of the older and 90% of the younger children are engaging in moderate-to-vigorous activity on a regular basis. The younger children (NCYFS II) spend 3 kcal/min/kg daily. The most recent Youth Risk Behaviour Survey disclosed that only 37% of adolescents spend more than 20 min/day in vigorous activity.

Oja then returned to Riddoch and Boreham who reviewed the literature on studies of children's heart rate as measure of intensity of exercise. They found that in generating heart rates of 120–140/min (30–50% of $VO_{2\,max}$) children were exercising from 40 to 110 min/day, depending on the study. For exercise of moderate intensity (HR of 150–169) (60–80% of $VO_{2\,max}$) children were exercising for 15–40 min/day. To attain heart rates ≥ 170 (90% of $VO_{2\,max}$) children were exercising for 5–20 min/day, depending on the study. These results are consistent with each other. On the other hand, ascertaining the prevalence of sufficiently active children is highly dependent on the threshold chosen:

If 20 min @ HR > 159 three times a week, then 0% of children will be found to be fit. But if set at 10 min @ HR > 139 three times a week, then 46% of children will be considered acceptably fit.

In conclusion, Oja said that the large majority of children are acceptably active using adult standards for activity. However, since children are generally much more active than adults, specific standards of childhood activity are needed. Another unanswered question is whether or not children's free-play activities are healthy. It is to be deplored, as noted by Sallis, that the mean yearly decline in activity level is 2.7% in postpubertal boys and 7.5% in postpubertal girls.

Oja's exercise prescription is that all adolescents should be physically active nearly every day and at a minimum should exercise three or more times a week for 20 min at a time. Oja also pointed out that there is no hard evidence that fitness has declined in American youth other than the prevalence of obesity, which increased 54% among 6 to 11-year-old children from 1960 to 1990 and 39% in 12 to 17-year-old adolescents over the same period of time.

Oja concluded that we need more research on the effects of various levels of fitness on health benefits. In terms of public policy we do not yet know the numbers of children who are actually at increased risk. He also concluded that good health in childhood facilitates good health in adults and that decreased activity and fitness in childhood may lead to compromised adult health. Finally, he noted that exercise in childhood is health-promoting behavior. We need to gather more information and to set clear standards for fitness so that similar studies can be done in many countries with robust and comparable outcomes.

Rontoyannis noted that one-third of the Greek population live in Athens and that 30% of them are under 20 years of age. Because of crowded urban conditions it is becoming more and more difficult to find free places to play. Therefore, physical education (PE) classes are the only chance left to indulge in active play. Currently, PE classes meet for only 2–3 h per week. Most of the activity in PE class involves motor-cognitive rather than aerobic activity. Therefore, Athenian youth suffer from hypokinesia, which has been linked to atherosclerosis in adulthood.

Rontoyannis continued by describing the results of a prospective study he did of an especially energetic program of PE for adolescents; 160 students of both sexes participated. Group one had 3 h/week of standard PE. Group 2 had an extra 4–8 h/week of energetic ball playing in addition to the standard PE. Dr. Rontoyannis noted transient improvements in several proxy risk factors for ASCVD including decreased TC/HDL-C ratio and increased $ApoA_1$/ApoB ratio, as well as decreased skinfold thickness. He concluded that there is evidence that intense and prolonged playground activity leads to favorable changes in aerobic power and proxy measures of ASCVD. However, these changes were not seen consistently in both sexes, nor did they persist for 18 months when a subgroup was retested. More research needs to be done on changes in such proxy measures as well as to ascertain the molecular mechanisms that generate the observed effects and their transience.

Stallings then presented the results of a recent study she performed in 34 prepubertal obese and nonobese black and white children, 5–12 years old, in an attempt to elucidate the reason for the epidemic of obesity among black preadolescents and adolescents. Of all the parameters studied FFM and ethnic group were the only significant predictors of resting energy expenditure which was lower in black children than in white children ($1,312 \pm 38$ vs. $1,524 \pm 43$ kcal/ day). She found no differences in any measure of fitness. The only metabolic marker that differed significantly between the races was fasting serum glucose which was 77 ± 13 mg/dl in black children and 85 ± 7 mg/dl in white children. These findings may provide information on the pathophysiology of childhood obesity in different races in the USA and may suggest treatment strategies to counteract the lower resting energy expenditure in black children.

Grave summarized the results of studies performed by Cooper and his colleagues at Harbor-UCLA Medical Center that were funded by a grant from the National Institutes of Health. Cooper studied the effects of a 5-week program of aerobic exercise training in 44 adolescent girls randomized either to a control situation of classroom learning about exercise physiology or to a similar learning program plus 2 h of ergometric training per day 5 days a week for 5 weeks. Cooper found that the girls who exercised increased their femoral muscle mass by a mean of 4% and their $VO_{2\,max}$ by a mean of 12%. The least fit girls improved their $VO_{2\,max}$ most, a relationhip characterized by a statistical method of best fit. Cooper also found that serum osteocalcin levels in the exercised girls increased by a mean of 39% at the end of 5 weeks. Osteocalcin is a vitamin K-dependent bone protein that serves as a marker for new bone formation. Cooper also found increase in serum levels of IGF-I, GH, and GHBP in the girls who exercised that were proportional to increases in their femoral muscle mass.

The challenge that Cooper's work presents is to incorporate a similar long-term exercise program into adolescent girls' lifestyles. Instead of shunning PE and school sports programs girls should welcome the opportunity to become healthier and more physically fit. By exercising their muscles, their bones will become denser and stronger, an improvement which will last a lifetime and which will decrease their future risk of osteoporosis.

Both adolescent boys and adolescent girls become progressively unfit as they get older. By the time they are seniors in high school 56% of boys and 70% of girls fail to engage in vigorous physical activity at least 3 times/week by self-report (Sallis). Cooper has documented that this gender difference in activity has made American girls less fit than American boys of the same age and strikingly less fit than Scandinavian girls tested by Åstrand in 1952. The mean $VO_{2\,max}$ of the American girls in 1984 and 1995 was nearly 1 liter/min less than their Scandinavian counterparts. The $VO_{2\,max}$ of the American boys, by contrast, nearly equaled that of the Scandinavian boys tested by Åstrand in 1952.

These decreases in physical activity and fitness may explain most of the recent epidemic of obesity among American girls in their second decade. Data from the HANES III show that obesity in adolescent girls has increased from 5 to 15% in African American and Hispanic populations over the past 20 years. Although the prevalence of obese boys has also increased over the past 20 years, the problem is more alarming among the girls. Girls actively try to avoid physical education classes and other sports activity for fear of seeming 'uncool' and from a mistaken idea of being accepted by peers and 'fitting in' as their highest priority, to the detriment of their current physical fitness and their future health.

Gilman D. Grave, MD, National Institute of Child Health and Human Development, National Institutes of Health, Bethesda, MD 20852 (USA)

Simopoulos AP (ed): Nutrition and Fitness: Evolutionary Aspects, Children's Health,
Programs and Policies. World Rev Nutr Diet. Basel, Karger, 1997, vol 81, pp 90–97

....

Nutritional Needs of the Exercising Child

Virginia A. Stallings

Division of Gastroenterology and Nutrition, Children's Hospital of Philadelphia,
Department of Pediatrics, University of Pennsylvania School of Medicine,
Philadelphia, Pa., USA

In many countries and cultures, participation in individual or team athletics begins at an early age. Yet unlike adults, the young athlete must meet the nutritional needs for optimal growth, body composition and pubertal development as well as those for participation in the chosen sport. Various sports-related nutritional practices which are common in the adult world of athletics are often inappropriately applied by the parent or coach to the growing child or adolescent who is more vulnerable to the possible negative effects of dietary manipulation. There are diverse benefits for the child who participates in regular general physical exercise and/or organized athletic activities, such as enjoyment, improved health, fitness and motor skills, and psychosocial development including positive social interactions and improved self-esteem. The parents and coaches of young athletes, and to some extent the athletes themselves, must understand the interactions of normal growth and development, and the special nutritional and fluid needs of children to allow them to create a pattern of dietary intake which supports both the needs for growth and for athletic performance.

There are other issues which indirectly affect the nutritional decisions of children who are participating in organized sport. The economic, regional, educational and cultural environment of the parents, coaches and children influence the usual food/nutrient intake patterns, and the more specific food practices related to athletic performance. In addition, the level of commitment of the parents, coaches and child athlete to achieve a high level of performance in competition, a focus on winning rather than on participation, may be associated with implementation of inappropriate nutritional practices for the young athlete in an effort to gain a competitive advantage.

Nutritional Issues

Nutritional issues for the exercising child are primarily in three areas: adequate energy intake to ensure optimal growth, body composition and pubertal development, in addition to energy intake for increased physical activity; adequate intake of dietary iron and calcium, which are the micronutrients generally at-risk for poor intake in children; and increased fluid needs for young competitive and recreational athletes.

Energy Needs

The definition of energy balance, as stated by the World Health Organization (WHO) [1], is 'the level of energy intake that will balance energy expenditure when the individual has a body size and composition, and a level of physical activity consistent with long-term good health. In children..., the energy requirement includes the energy needs associated with the deposition of tissues (growth) ... at rates consistent with good health'. So, for children and adolescents, the goal is to provide energy to achieve normal growth at the individual child's genetic potential, normal body composition (optimal proportions of muscle, bone and fat), and to maintain normal patterns of activities of daily living including the extra energy demands for athletic activities. Negative energy balance (semistarvation) results in alteration of all these desirable goals, and leads to abnormal patterns of growth and body composition, decreased physical activity and suboptimal athletic performance. Persistent excess positive energy balance also fails to meet these goals and results in more rapid growth rates, abnormal body composition (excess adiposity or obesity) and decreased physical activity and suboptimal athletic performance.

Recommendations and Equations

Various sources in the literature provide tables of the predicted total daily energy needs for groups of healthy, normally grown children, with the Recommended Dietary Allowances (RDA) [2] being the standard for the United States (table 1). Yet in the practice of sports medicine and nutrition, the coaches and parents want to know the energy requirement of the young athlete to achieve a normal pattern of body composition, growth, pubertal development and the greater than usual level of physical activity. The estimate of the energy requirement is then translated into a food intake pattern that is compatible with the young athlete's personal and family food preferences and practices.

The alternative to the population-based recommendations (the RDA approach) for energy intake is to use one of the various mathematical formulas to predict the basal metabolic rate or resting energy expenditure (REE, the

Table 1. Energy intake recommendation from the recommended dietary allowances (10th edition) with median heights and weights

Category	Age	Weight kg	Height cm	REE kcal/day	Average energy allowance, kcal		
					multiples of REE	per kg	per day
Infants	0.0–0.5	6	60	320	2.03	108	650
	0.5–1.0	9	71	500	1.70	98	850
Children	1–3	13	90	740	1.76	102	1,300
	4–6	20	112	950	1.89	90	1,800
	7–10	28	132	1,130	1.77	70	2,000
Males	11–14	45	157	1,440	1.70	55	2,500
	15–18	66	176	1,760	1.67	45	3,000
	19–24	72	177	1,780	1.67	40	2,900
Females	11–14	46	157	1,310	1.67	47	2,200
	15–18	55	163	1,370	1.60	40	2,200
	19–24	58	164	1,350	1.60	38	2,200

term that will be used here), and then adjust the REE with sets of physical activity factors reflecting the child or adolescents' usual practices to predict the total daily energy needs. The most commonly known method to estimate the REE needs is the Harris and Benedict [3] equations for adults which uses the subject's gender, age, height and weight to estimate the REE. These equations were derived mostly from adult measurements (including some infants, no children or adolescents) and is not recommended for use in the pediatric age group. More recently, the WHO created new REE prediction equations which are designed for use in infants, children and adolescents, and are shown in table 2. These equations use the child's age group, gender and body weight to predict REE, and are the equations used in clinical practice in many pediatric care settings. A more detailed evaluation of the WHO data resulted in the Schofield [4] equations, which provide predictive equations for REE using either weight alone, or weight and height (table 3), and age group and gender. Still, the energy needs of an individual child athlete are difficult to predict due to the variations in metabolic demands of alterations in growth, body composition, and the extra energy needs for athletic training and competition. Measurement of REE is the best available method to accurately determine the individual's energy needs for use in both clinical and sports medicine to promote weight gain or loss, or to provide for weight maintenance.

Table 2. WHO equations for predicting resting energy expenditure from body weight (W), gender and age group

Age range years	kcal/day
Males	
0–3	$60.9W - 54$
3–10	$22.7W + 495$
10–18	$17.5W + 651$
18–30	$15.3W + 679$
Females	
0–3	$61.0W - 51$
3–10	$22.5W + 499$
10–18	$12.2W + 746$
18–30	$14.7W + 496$

Table 3. Schofield equations for predicting resting energy expenditure from body weight (W), height (H), gender and age group

Age range years	kcal/day
Males	
0–3	$0.167W + 1517.4H - 617.6$
3–10	$19.59W + 130.3H + 414.9$
10–18	$16.25W + 137.2H + 515.5$
18–30	$15.057W + 10.04H + 705.8$
Females	
0–3	$16.252W + 1023.2H - 413.5$
3–10	$16.969W + 161.8H + 371.2$
10–18	$8.365W + 465.0H + 200.0$
18–30	$13.623W + 283.0H + 98.2$

Resting Energy Expenditure by Indirect Calorimetry

The study of energy metabolism in clinical and sports settings has been possible in recent years due to the advances in the construction of the open-circuit ventilated-hood indirect calorimeters. The indirect calorimeter or metabolic cart measures oxygen consumption and carbon dioxide production by the subject, and these values are used to calculate the REE expressed as kilocalories or kilojoules per day. The REE measurement should be conducted under standardized conditions to ensure the accuracy of the data and clinical interpretation. The optimal REE measurement is conducted in a supine, resting, but awake, subject in the early morning (0.700–10.00 h), after a night of

Table 4. Approximate energy expenditure for various activities in relation to resting needs for males and females of average size[1]

Activity category[2]	Representative value for activity factor per unit of time activity
Resting Sleeping, reclining	REE × 1.0
Very light Seated and standing activities, painting trades, driving, laboratory work, typing, sewing, ironing, cooking, playing cards, playing a musical instrument	REE × 1.5
Light Walking on a level surface at 2.5–3 mph, garage work, electrical trades, carpentry, restaurant trades, house-cleaning, child care, golf, sailing, table tennis	REE × 2.5
Moderate Walking 3.5–4 mph, weeding and hoeing, carrying a load, cycling, skiing, tennis, dancing	REE × 5.0
Heavy Walking with load uphill, tree felling, heavy manual digging, basketball, climbing, football, soccer	REE × 7.0

[1] Based on values reported by Durnin and Passmore [6] and WHO [1].
[2] When reported as multiples of basal needs, the expenditures of males and females are similar.

restful sleep, an overnight fast, and prior to any physical activity or meta-bolically active medications (known to change the heart rate, i.e. bronchodi-lators). The usual clinical REE lasts 30–60 min, with the first 10 min omitted from data analysis to account for subject equilibration.

Today, REE is measured to determine the total energy needs of an individual subject to achieve a specific nutritional goal (weight maintenance, loss or gain). To estimate the total daily energy requirements of a subject from the measurement of the REE over 1 h requires further calculations, and an understanding of the components of daily total energy expenditure (TEE). REE represents a large portion of the energy needed each day. The additional energy needed for normal growth and physical activity (everything except quietly resting supine), or support therapeutic growth acceleration must be added to the REE to determine TEE. Table 4 shows the physical activity

Table 5. Estimated energy needs for competitive swimmers (kcal)

Age years	REE		Total	
	male	female	male	female
<10	2,000	1,800	2,200–2,900	2,000–2,800
11–14	2,500	2,200	2,700–3,600	2,400–3,200
15–18	3,000	2,200	3,200–4,000	2,400–3,500
19–22	2,900	2,000	3,100–4,200	2,200–3,700

and usual growth factors for healthy, normally active children [2]. They range from 1.70 to $2.03 \times$ REE based upon the age and gender group. Children who are significantly more physically active will require more energy. For example, Berning [5] has estimated the increased energy expenditure and requirements for children and young adults participating in competitive swimming, as shown in table 5. Similar data are needed to estimate the energy expended by children and adolescent athletes in various individual and team sports.

The last consideration in using REE to determine the total daily energy requirement is to add a factor which adjusts for 'catch-up' growth when indicated. As previously discussed, the REE is adjusted by a factor (1.70 to $2.07 \times$ REE) that provides adequate energy for the usual amount of weight gain and usual physical activity in healthy children. In some children, the goal may be to increase the rate of weight gain above the normal rate and this requires additional energy (as well as other nutrients). A general approach is to use the approximate relationship that 1 kg of weight gain (or loss) requires an excess (or deficiency) of 7,700 calories. In pounds, the relationship is one pound to 3,500 cal. If 1 kg weight gain is planned to occur over 1 month, then 7,700 kcal ÷ 30 days/month = 257 kcal/day additional calories to be added to the previously calculated total caloric intake goal. If 1 kg weight gain is to be achieved over 14 days, then 513 kcal/day (7,700 kcal ÷ 14 days) are added to the total caloric intake goal.

Nonenergy Nutrients

Once the energy requirements of young, growing athletes have been met by the consumption of a broad variety of food, the requirements for protein, carbohydrate and the micronutrients generally are met. Note that the usual intake of protein by US children and adolescents significantly exceeds the recommendations by 50–100%, so there is no need to specifically recommend a higher protein diet. Since dietary iron and calcium intake are often sub-optimal in children and adolescents, intake of these nutrients should be evaluated, particularly in children who have a limited set of food preferences. The vegetarian athlete will have limited access to dietary iron, and supplementation should be considered. Iron deficiency anemia will decrease both the cognitive and athletic performance of the child athlete, and should be screened for by laboratory tests (hemoglobin or hematocrit) in high-risk athletes and treated when it occurs. The young athlete who is lactose intoler-ant and does not ingest dairy products with lactase enzyme supplements will have limited access to dietary calcium, and supplementation should be considered. Since the majority of the adult peak bone mass is acquired during childhood and adolescence, providing optimal calcium intake during these years is of lifelong importance. Screening for the effects of chronically poor dietary calcium intake is more complex than that for iron deficiency anemia. Yet, the development and availability of the dual-energy X-ray ab-sorptiometry (DEXA) technology make screening for osteopenia and osteo-porosis possible. Young athletes whose primary sport does not require full weight bearing, such as swimming, are more at-risk for a relative decrease in the usual advantage of physical activity enhancing bone mineralization during childhood.

Fluid Needs

In general, child athletes are considered to be more at-risk for dehydra-tion than their adult counterparts. Children are more effected by heat stress and produce less sweat in response to environmental heat. In addition, children have a physiological background including a lower cardiac output and higher baseline body temperature. The child athlete is also less aware of his/her state of hydration, and less likely to have an appropriate level of thirst for the level of dehydration. Consequently, coach or parental supervi-sion of fluid intake is required to keep the young athlete well hydrated throughout the periods of training and competition. As with most athletes, children will consume more total fluids if the fluids are cool and flavored. The use of diluted fruit drinks, rather than the sport drinks which have been designed for adult needs, have been suggested, as well as the avoidance of carbonated or caffeinated beverages. Particular supervisory attention needs to be provided for the young athlete whose sports require significant protec-tive gear during warm weather training and competition, and to young swimmers who often are unaware of sweating and the need to consume adequate fluids.

Conclusion

Not only does participation in athletic activities have many advantages for children, it also may expose them to suboptimal nutrition-related health practices common to the world of adult athletics. Parents, coaches, and to some extent the young athlete, must understand the special nutritional needs of the child and adolescent, and need to recognize and avoid risky nutritional practices, and embrace and implement sound practices. Life-long attitudes and habits about food, health and physical activity are formed during childhood. Coaches and parents, as well as elite athletes and the sports media, are the powerful influences who provide the majority of the nutrition and health facts to the child and adolescent. The child athlete requires few specialized nutritional practices, other than to ensure that he/she receives adequate energy intake which is provided by a variety of foods, to allow optimal growth, body composition and pubertal development, and to allow optimal participation in athletic activities.

References

1   FAO/WHO/UNU Expert Consultation, Energy and Protein Requirements. Geneva, World Health Organization, 1985, pp 71–112.
2   National Academy of Sciences, Recommended Dietary Allowances. Washington, National Academy Press, 1989, pp 24–38.
3   Harris JA, Benedict FG: A Biometric Study of Basal Metabolism in Man. Washington, Carnegie Institution, 1919, publ 279.
4   Schofield WN: Predicting basal metabolic rate, new standards and review of previous work. Hum Nutr Clin Nutr 1985;39c(is):5–42.
5   Berning JR: Nutritional concerns of recreational endurance athletes with an emphasis on swimming; in Ratzin Jackson CG (ed): Nutrition for the Recreational Athlete. Boca Raton, CRC Press, 1994, pp 37–53.
6   Durnin JVGA, Passmore R: Energy, Work and Leisure. London, Heinemann Educational Books, 1967, pp 1–166.

Virginia A. Stallings, MD, Division of Gastroenterology and Nutrition,
Children's Hospital of Philadelphia, 34th Street and Civic Center Blvd.,
Philadelphia, PA 19104 (USA)

Simopoulos AP (ed): Nutrition and Fitness: Evolutionary Aspects, Children's Health, Programs and Policies. World Rev Nutr Diet. Basel, Karger, 1997, vol 81, pp 98–104

....

Health-Related Physical Activity and Fitness among European Children and Adolescents

Pekka Oja

UKK Institute for Health Promotion Research, Tampere, Finland

The role of physical activity in the promotion of adult health has been subject to intensive scientific interest during the 1990s [1, 2]. The current evidence is convincing enough to have warranted authoritative recommendations for physical activity to be included in public health policies [3–7].

Only recently have the public health implications of children's and adolescents' exercise and fitness been systematically evaluated [8–11]. According to the general framework of Blair et al. [12] there are complex interrelationships between childhood exercise and fitness, childhood health, adult exercise and fitness, and adult health. Although presently there is no good prospective evidence to show that health in adult years is directly linked with exercise and fitness in childhood and adolescence, exercise and fitness in early years can promote adult health also by enhancing health in childhood and by preparing children for life-time regular physical activity. These potential long-term health consequences highlight the public health importance of children's exercise and fitness.

This paper reviews briefly the current knowledge on the relationship between exercise, fitness, and health in childhood, and the status of children's health-related exercise and fitness with particular focus on the European situation. For brevity the terms children and childhood cover both children and adolescents, if not otherwise indicated. Childhood refers to the period until the start of puberty and adolescence starts with puberty and ends with adulthood. The term exercise is used to cover widely all types of physical activity.

Childhood Exercise and Fitness vs. Childhood Health

Several comprehensive reviews have been published during the 1990s on the health effects of childhood exercise [8, 9, 13–15]. These reviews serve as the basis for the following brief overview, which focuses on the most frequently studied health outcomes, namely coronary heart disease (CHD) risk factors, obesity, and bone density and mass.

Cross-sectional studies indicate that active and fit children tend to have a more favorable CHD risk profile than sedentary and unfit children. Resting blood pressure is lower in children with high aerobic fitness and this difference is seen from age 5 on. Physically active and fit children also have a more favorable lipoprotein profile with respect to triglycerides and HDL-cholesterol. Results of prospective studies are less consistent providing little evidence that in healthy children enhanced physical activity reduces the risk probably because initial low risk is unlikely to drop. Many of the longitudinal studies are also plagued by preselection and relatively short interventions. It appears that whatever CHD risk reduction occurs seems to affect children at high risk.

Obesity is the most common pediatric illness in many Western countries and thus a major public health challenge. Training studies indicate that exercise can induce at least a short-term reduction in body fat of obese children and adolescents. Exercise may increase the daily metabolic rate more than the approximately 10% increase expected from the activity itself reflecting the possible enhancement of basal metabolic rate. There are impressive recent results of long-term interventions combining exercise, low-calorie diet and behavioral modification in preventing the development of childhood obesity. Epstein et al. [16] showed that in 10 years one-third of obese children had decreased the percentage overweight by 20% or more, and 30% were no longer obese.

Several, although not all, cross-sectional studies have shown a positive relationship between habitual physical activity and bone density or mass in children. Kannus et al. [17] showed a consistent playing-to-nonplaying arm difference of humeral shaft mineral density between young tennis players and controls. The difference was the larger, up to 23%, the earlier the playing was started with a noticeable drop in the effect when the playing was started after the menarche. There appears to be a threshold of effective activity beyond which a mineral loss may occur as seen in female athletes and ballet dancers.

In summary, mostly cross-sectional evidence is consistent with the hypothesis that regular exercise and good fitness are linked with beneficial disease risk profile in terms of CHD risk factors, such as elevated blood pressure and atherogenic lipoprotein profile, obesity and bone loss.

Health-Related Physical Activity in Children

How active are today's children with respect to health? This simple question is difficult to answer, because there are no commonly accepted criteria for health-enhancing physical activity specific for children and studies have used different criteria usually derived from information on adults. Two types of studies, those based on self-reporting and those on heart rate (HR) measurement, provide partial evidence.

Self-Report Studies

Riddoch and Boreham [18] recently reviewed the relevant, mostly European, self-report studies on physical activity habits of children. According to these studies the mean time spent on sports, leisure and other physical activities by children varied from 30 to 80 min/day. These mean values are above the guideline suggested by Blair et al. [12] as sufficient for health benefits.

Assessment of the proportion of sufficiently active children yielded widely variable (10–80%) figures depending on the criteria used in these studies. Based on selected large nationally representative studies Riddoch and Boreham [18] appraised it to be about 60–70% of all children. In comparison, 3/4 of Canadian children [19] and about 90% of American children [12] have been estimated to be sufficiently active according to self-reporting.

The self-report studies indicate consistently that activity declines with age after the peak at age around 13–14 years, and boys are more active than girls at all ages. According to Sallis [20] the mean difference between boys and girls is approximately 14%, and the mean yearly decline 2% for boys and 2.5% for girls.

Heart Rate Studies

Riddoch and Boreham [18] located over 20 studies on children's physical activity as measured by HR monitoring. These studies covered both boys and girls between the ages of 3 and 18 years. The data of the studies were classified into 3 groups: low-intensity activity, 30–50% $\dot{V}O_{2max} = HR$ 120–149; moderate intensity activity, 50–70% $\dot{V}O_{2max} = HR$ 150–169; high intensity activity, $>70\%$ $\dot{V}O_{2max} = HR > 169$. According to this classification the mean daily activity times in the reported studies were 40–110 min/day at low intensity, 15–40 min/day at moderate intensity, and 5–20 min/day at high intensity.

In two studies [21, 22] reviewed by Riddoch and Boreham [18] the percentage of children participating in physical activity promoting cardiopulmonary fitness was reported. According to a rigid criterion (3 times per week × 20 min at HR > 159) none of the children were active enough. A more modest criterion (3 × 10 min at HR > 139) showed 46% of the children to be active.

The HR studies also show boys to be more active than girls. The difference is considerable at high-intensity activities, but is reduced at low-intensity activities.

Overall Picture of Children's Activity

There is a large discrepancy between the self-report and the HR studies with respect to the proportion of sufficiently active children. While the former suggest the majority (60–90%) of Western children to be active, the latter seem to suggest a much lower figure, perhaps below 50%. Considering that self-reporting is known to yield overestimation and the heart-rate assessment takes into account mainly the aerobically effective activity, thus omitting health benefits accrued through other mechanisms, the true percentage is likely to be between these figures.

In estimating the long-term health consequences of childhood activity it is important to keep in mind that physical activity declines steadily not only from childhood to adolescence but also from adolescence to adulthood. Thus, while a large proportion of today's children seem to be active in a way that if maintained into adult life, health benefits would be conferred, a considerable proportion is insufficiently active already during childhood and adolescence. A group at particularly high risk of inactivity is that of aging adolescent girls.

What Kind of Exercise for Children and Adolescents?

What kind and how much physical activity is beneficial for the health of children and adolescents? According to an international consensus group [10] adolescents should (1) be physically active daily or nearly every day ..., and (2) engage in three or more sessions per week of activities that last 20 min or more at a time and that require moderate-to-vigorous levels of exertion.

In the absence of specific health exercise criteria for children, these and other [23] recommendations remain to be based on adult criteria. They emphasize aerobic training with continuous bouts of moderate-to-vigorous exercise. This does not confer very well with children's natural play-like activity, which is typically sporadic, diverse and intermittent and takes place daily [24]. Obviously, there is an urgent need for more research in establishing specific health-enhancing exercise criteria for children.

Health-Related Physical Fitness of Children

There is a large amount of normative data on children's fitness from North America, Europe and Australia. In Europe the EUROFIT test battery of physical fitness [25] has been employed in many countries, but lack of health criteria norms make the health-related interpretation of this information virtually impossible. What is known, is that boys are clearly fitter, up to 25%, than girls and while fitness remains quite stable among boys with aging, the girl's fitness declines steadily, approximately 2.2% per year, from late childhood on [20]. This information again highlights the increased activity-related risk among aging girls.

There is an often expressed concern that youth fitness has declined during the past decades [26–30]. There is no solid evidence to verify this except for obesity. The prevalence of youth obesity has increased in the USA from 1960 to 1990 by 54% in 6–11 year olds and by 39% in 12–17 year olds. These figures strongly suggest that also the obesity–related performance capabilities such as weight-related aerobic power and weight-bearing muscle performance may have declined.

Conclusions

Research evidence suggests that (1) childhood exercise and good fitness are beneficial for health already in childhood; (2) inactivity in childhood is likely to lead to increased risk of hypokinetic diseases in adulthood; (3) childhood activity and good fitness can lead to life-time adoption of regular activity, and (4) exercise during adulthood is definitely a health-enhancing behavior. Thus, the promotion of health-related physical activity and fitness among children and adolescents can have tremendous impact on public health.

However, we know insufficiently how many youth are at increased risk because of inactivity and poor fitness, and what are the exact properties of health-enhancing physical activity for children. Therefore, in order to guide public health policies, it is vitally important for the research community to (1) develop and standardize valid, reliable and practical measuring tools for the assessment of health-related activity and fitness of children; (2) develop health-related criteria norms of activity and fitness specific for children, and (3) provide accurate information on the status and trends of childhood activity and fitness.

References

1   Bouchard C, Shephard RJ, Stephens T (eds): Physical Activity, Fitness, and Health. International Proceedings and Consensus Statement. Champaign, Human Kinetics, 1994.
2   Vuori I, Fentem P: The significance of sport for society; Health. Council of Europe, Committee for the Development of Sport. Council of Europe Press, 1995.

3   American College of Sports Medicine: Position stand. Physical activity, physical fitness, and hypertension. Med Sci Sports Exerc 1993;25:i-x.
4   Centers for Disease Control and Prevention and the American College of Sports Medicine: Physical activity and public health. A recommendation from the Centers for Disease Control and Prevention and the American College of Sports Medicine. JAMA 1995;273:402–406.
5   Council of Europe: 8th Conference of European Ministers Responsible for Sport. Strasbourg, 1995.
6   World Health Organization (WHO) and Federation of Sports Medicine (FIMS) Committee on Physical Activity for Health: Exercise for health. Bull WHO 1995;73:135–136.
7   Research Quarterly for Exercise and Sport: Physical activity, health, and well-being. An International Scientific Consensus Conference. Res Q Exerc Sport 1995:66.
8   Nelson MA: The role of physical education and children's activity in the public health. Res Q Exerc Sport 1991;62:148–150.
9   Sallis JF, McKenzie TL: Physical education's role in public health. Res Q Exerc Sport 1991;62: 124–137.
10   Sallis JF, Patrick K: Physical activity guidelines for adolescents: Consensus statement. Pediatr Exerc Sci 1994;6:302–314.
11   Trippe H: Children and sport. Br Med J 1996;312:199.
12   Blair SN, Clark DB, Cureton KJ, Powell KE: Exercise and fitness in childhood: Implications for a lifetime of health; in Gisolfi CV, Lamb DL (eds): Perspectives in Exercise Science and Sports Medicine. Youth, Exercise and Sport. Indianapolis, Benchmark Press, 1989, vol 2, pp 401–430.
13   Malina RM: Growth, exercise, fitness, and later outcomes; in Bouchard C, Shephard RJ, Stephens T, Sutton JR, McPherson BD (eds): Exercise, Fitness, and Health: A Consensus of Current Knowledge. Champaign, Human Kinetics, 1990, pp 637–653.
14   Baranowski T, Bouchard C, Bar-Or O, Bricker T, Heath G, Kim SYS, Malina R, Obarzanek E, Pate R, Strong WB, Truman B, Washington R: Assessment, prevalence, and cardiovascular benefits of physical activity and fitness in youth. Med Sci Sports Exerc 1992;24:S237–S247.
15   Bar-Or O: Childhood and adolescent physical activity and fitness and adult risk profile; in Bouchard C, Shephard RJ, Stephens T (eds): Physical Activity, Fitness, and Health. Campaign, Human Kinetics, 1994, pp 931–942.
16   Epstein LH, Valoski A, Wing RR, McCurley J: Ten-year outcomes of behavioral family-based treatment for childhood obesity. Health Psychol 1994;13:373–383.
17   Kannus P, Haapasalo H, Sankelo M, Sievänen H, Pasanen M, Heinonen A, Oja P, Vuori I: Effect of starting age of physical activity on bone mass in the dominant arm of tennis and squash players. Ann Intern Med 1995;123:27–31.
18   Riddoch CJ, Boreham CAG: The health-related physical activity of children. Sports Med 1995;19: 86–102.
19   Shephard RJ: Fitness of a nation: Lessons from the Canada Fitness Survey. Med Sport Sci 1986; 22:116–131.
20   Sallis JF: Epidemiology of physical activity and fitness in children and adolescents. Crit Rev Food Sci Nutr 1993;33:403–408.
21   Armstrong N, Williams J, Balding J, Gentle P, Kirby B: Cardiopulmonary fitness, physical activity patterns, and selected coronary risk factor variables in 11–16-year-olds. Pediatr Exerc Sci 1991;3: 219–228.
22   Armstrong N, Bray S: Physical activity patterns defined by continuous heart rate monitoring. Arch Dis Child 1991;66:245–247.
23   Strong WB, Deckelbaum RJ, Gidding SS, Kavey R-EV, Washington R, Willmore JH, Perry CL: Integrated cardiovascular health promotion in childhood: A statement for health professionals from the subcommittee on artherosclerosis and hypertension in childhood of the Council on Cardiovascular Disease in the Young, American Heart Association. AHA Medical/Scientific Statement. Special Report, 1992.
24   Cale L, Harris J: Exercise recommendations for children and young people. Phys Educ Rev 1993; 16:89–98.
25   Council of Europe, Committee for the Development of Sport, Committee of Experts on Sports Research: Eurofit. Handbook for the Eurofit tests of physical fitness. Rome, 1988.

26 American College of Sports Medicine: Opinion statement on physical fitness in children and youth. Med Sci Sports Exerc 1988;20:422–423.
27 Blair SN: Are American children and youth fit? The need for better data. Res Q Exerc Sport 1992; 63:120–123.
28 Corbin CB, Pangrazi RP: Are American children and youth fit? Res Q Exerc Sport 1992;63:96–106.
29 The Lancet: Editorials. Young and unfit? 1992;340:19–20
30 Kuntzleman CT: Childhood fitness: What is happening? What needs to be done? Prev Med 1993; 22:520–532.

Pekka Oja, UKK Institute for Health Promotion Research,
PO Box 30, FIN–33501 Tampere (Finland)

Simopoulos AP (ed): Nutrition and Fitness: Evolutionary Aspects, Children's Health, Programs and Policies. World Rev Nutr Diet. Basel, Karger, 1997, vol 81, pp 105–107

....

Summary of Part 3

Peter G. Bourne

American Association for World Health, Washington, D.C., USA

Lee described the fragmented nature of programming and policy-making in the USA covering 50 states and more than 3,000 local authorities. While government could play an overall leadership role and conduct research, such as through the Centers for Disease Control and the National Center for Health Statistics, nonprofit organizations were usually the primary implementors.

He identified 6 areas where the Federal Government played a significant role:

(1) Public education and information: Working with the Department of Agriculture to develop educational material. Food supplement programs such as Women, Infant and Child Feeding (WIC). Working jointly with private groups. Providing information and leadership through The President's Council on Physical Fitness and Sports.

(2) Working with professional groups: The Coalition for Health and Fitness, with Health Maintenance organizations, and with physician's groups to put prevention into practice through education about nutrition and fitness.

(3) Food services: Developing dietary guidelines and monitoring dietary policy.

(4) Food safety: Monitoring food safety through food inspectors and more recently through more technologically advanced methods.

(5) Nutrition labeling: Giving people the information they needed to know in order to make healthy decisions including providing levels of salt content and additives.

(6) Research and surveillance: Supporting studies such as the classic Framingham study on heart disease, collating and disseminating research from a wide variety of sources and using it to shape policy.

Lee particularly identified the forthcoming Surgeon General's Report on Fitness and Health, to be released this summer as a key document in this area.

Chen emphasized that, in China, meeting basic caloric and protein needs was still a primary consideration. However, with improved economic circumstances this was now primarily a problem of isolated rural and mountain areas. The primary causes were poverty, unsanitary water supplies, lack of breast feeding, and sexual discrimination against female infants. Specific strategies were being implemented to address these problems including provision of vitamin A supplements and soy bean products to reduce anemia. An additional problem was now being posed by people's increasing appetite for meat, resulting in grain supplies being diverted for animal feed. The changing diet was resulting in an increase in the incidence of chronic disease. Educational efforts were directed at stressing the consumption of traditional foods, and controlling the eating of animal fat.

The government has recently launched a 'Sports for All' plan. There is a national commitment to improve sports and fitness emphasizing 'characteristic Chinese features'. The focus is on young people and popularizing a wide variety of sports.

The third speaker was Dr. Catherine Siandwazi of the Commonwealth Regional Health Community Secretariat for East, Central and Southern Africa. She stressed the declining nutrition situation in the region which had in the past affected mainly rural areas, but which was increasingly involving urban populations. The problems of vitamin A deficiency, iodine deficiency, anemia, and decreasing consumption of traditional foods were of particular concern. Her unit was established to assist governments in establishing nutrition programs, to train personnel, and in policy formulation. They also convened meetings of key government officials and other leaders to get commitment to support nutrition programs. Problems are being aggravated by a lack of resources and recurrent drought.

Matala described the historic interest in nutrition and fitness which underpins today's policies and programs in Greece. Following the reinstitution of the modern Olympic Games, the Greek government in 1899 passed legislation mandating recreational activity. Over the years the original components were changed, but physical education was built into the school curriculum. In the mid-1980s a 'Sports for All' movement was incorporated legislatively. An Office for Development of Sports was created in the Ministry of Culture. 7% of the population are currently involved. With changing diet patterns and lifestyle, Greeks, however, are today more obese and less fit than in previous decades.

What is now referred to as the 'Mediterranean diet' is essentially the Greek diet of the late 19th Century. That diet has changed significantly for the worse since 1960. Now there is a major educational effort to return people to the traditional diet. Although there is no equivalent to the FDA in Greece, there is a new level of interest in monitoring and improving food quality. Private institutions such as the Athens School of Public Health, the Department of Medicine at the University of Crete, and the Department of Nutrition and Dietetics at Harokopio are taking the lead in promoting interest in nutrition and health.

Van Mechelen addressed the European-wide context, especially the role of the Council of Europe and the European Commission. He described the 'Euro-Fit' Program which in two parts has established fitness standards and manuals for children and adults. Overall he felt Europeans had not done enough to establish programs and policies with no formal approval yet by member governments. He identified three publications by the Council of Europe on sports injuries, physical activity and the significance of sport for society.

Various food research studies had been conducted, but they were mainly epidemiological. The European Commission had published 'Nutrition and Cancer' but their other work tended to be similarly narrowly targeted. Now, however, there was an increasing move towards combining promotion of fitness and food.

The final speaker was Dr. Frank Katch of the US who proposed the creation of a new discipline 'exercise nutrition'. He suggested that nutrition and fitness needed to be combined together in academic institutions and placed not under departments of physical education or nutrition but in, perhaps, a school of life sciences.

A major theme that arose from the presentations was the clear distinction between the nutrition and fitness needs of developing nations as opposed to western industrialized societies. Meeting basic needs for calories, protein and micronutrients remains the primary objective for much of the world. Exercise is a secondary issue when the bulk of the population is of necessity involved in regular heavy labor. The problems of nutrition in developing countries and with some segments in the developed world remains one of overcoming poverty. In the affluent world where excessive calorie intake and sedentary lifestyle are the major problems, a completely different set of goals and national priorities involving education towards better eating habits and physical activity are necessary.

Peter G. Bourne, American Association for World Health,
2119 Leroy Place, NW, Washington, DC 20008 (USA)

Simopoulos AP (ed): Nutrition and Fitness: Evolutionary Aspects, Children's Health,
Programs and Policies. World Rev Nutr Diet. Basel, Karger, 1997, vol 81, pp 108–113

....

Nutrition and Physical Activity Perspectives for All Americans: Government and Private Sector Partnerships for the Twenty-First Century[1]

Philip R. Lee, Linda D. Meyers[2]

United States Department of Health and Human Services, Office of Public Health
and Science, Washington, D.C., USA

Americans have benefited from actions in public and private sectors to
ensure an abundant food supply and access to it, and to improve food safety,
update nutrition labeling, issue dietary recommendations and educate consumers and health professionals about their application, and conduct nutrition
research and surveillance. School lunch programs, Head Start and other public
assistant programs have nurtured millions. On the physical activity side, government and private sector initiatives have encouraged Americans to be more
physically active for health, performance in work or leisure pursuits, and safety.

As we face the many challenges remaining to fully achieve a healthy
citizenry, we are giving greater attention to collaboration among all levels of
government – Federal, state and local, and we are learning how to forge
partnerships and alliances with the private sector, both nonprofit and for-
profit. This presentation highlights a number of such efforts underway in the
United States to promote adoption of healthy dietary and physical activity

[1] Presented by P.R.L. at the Third International Conference on Nutrition and Fitness,
Athens, Greece, May 24–27, 1996, Session 6. National Programs and Policies Promoting
Better Nutrition, Physical Fitness and Sport for All.
[2] Drs. Lee and Meyers are from the Office of Public Health and Sciences in the United
States Department of Health and Human Services. Dr. Lee is Assistant Secretary for Health.
Dr. Meyers is Senior Nutrition Advisor, Office of Disease Prevention and Health Promotion.
The authors thank Dr. York Onnen for his many contributions to this presentation.

patterns. It is organized around activities directed toward public education, health professionals, food service, nutrition labeling, food safety, and research and surveillance.

Public Education and Information

As the impact of both science and demographics is felt, greater and more specific attention is being directed to subgroups in the population, to the elderly, to pregnant women, and to minorities. In addition, over the past decade consumer education efforts have become more innovative. The many uses of the Food Guide Pyramid and the Nutrition Facts label, including appearances by book character *Curious George,* are key examples of increased innovation. The US Department of Agriculture's (USDA) *Team Nutrition* initiative includes the use of two animated characters from the Disney film, *The Lion King,* to convey messages about healthy eating to children.

Collaboration is also increasing. For example, the new Alliance for the Dietary Guidelines is a partnership of food industry, health organizations and nutrition professional societies, with liaison representatives from government, who have joined together around the 1995 *Dietary Guidelines for Americans* to develop consumer-friendly messages consistent with the *Guidelines.* The National Coalition for Promoting Physical Activity is another example. Led by the American College of Sports Medicine, the American Alliance for Health, Physical Education, and Dance, and the American Heart Association, this group works with a range of public and private associations to increase public awareness, provide an opportunity to form partnerships, and to enhance delivery of consistent messages about physical activity.

Over the past decade, the government has strengthened its consumer education initiatives. There are now a number of activities throughout the Public Health Service within the Department of Health and Human Services, many of them involving collaborative efforts with the private sector or other governmental levels. Public education programs at the National Institutes of Health (NIH) revolve around specific disease risk-reduction programs, but have broader application and benefit. The National 5-A-Day for Better Health Program is a prominent example. Sponsored by the National Cancer Institute (NCI) with the Produce for Better Health Foundation, the program encourages Americans to eat five or more servings of fruits and vegetables every day. It is the largest public/private enterprise ever undertaken by the NCI and a model of collaboration. Since 1985, the National Cholesterol Education Program of the NIH's National Heart, Lung, and Blood Institute (NHLBI) has targeted health-care providers, patients, and the general public to increase awareness about the significance of lowering blood cholesterol levels through diet and physical activity as a means of preventing cardiovascular disease. More recently, and in recognition of the increasing prevalence of overweight in the United States, in 1994, the National Institute of Diabetes and Digestive and Kidney Diseases established the Weight-Control Information Network to foster transfer of scientific knowledge about obesity to patients, health professionals, and the general public.

The Centers for Disease Control and Prevention (CDC) recently embarked on the Nutrition and Physical Activity Communication initiative to promote physical activity and healthy eating among Americans. PAN – physical activity and nutrition – has just been initiated. It is a collaborative effort with the International Life Sciences Institute and Emory University that seeks to improve nutrition and physical activity practices among children. The CDC has also established physical activity guidelines for young people.

The President's Council on Physical Fitness and Sports has a long tradition of building partnerships with industry and promoting opportunities in physical activity, fitness, and sports for all Americans through information dissemination and public awareness about the importance of physical activity and fitness. A new Youth Fitness Campaign developed in collaboration with the Advertising Council is one example. Other education activities include the Nolan Ryan Fitness Guide, the Olympic IZZY promotion of fitness for all, the school-based President's Challenge Physical Fitness Awards Program, and the Healthy American Fitness Leaders recognition program and the Silver Eagle Corporation Program for Older Americans.

In the private sector, leadership organizations such as the American College of Sports Medicine, the American Dietetic Association, the American Heart Association, and the American Alliance for Health, Physical Education, Recreation and Dance are among a growing list of partners. Increasingly, other organizations are making themselves known as interested parties with the resources to make a difference at the community level. These include Boys and Girls Clubs of America, with over two thousand clubs, mostly in underserved areas; the National Park and Recreation Association, which recently launched the Beyond Fun and Games campaign in recognition of eroding support for public park and recreation resources; and the US National Senior Sports Organization, the officially recognized governing body for senior sports, which promotes the bi-annual Senior Olympics. Older adults ages 55 and above participate in a variety of sports for competition, fitness and camaraderie. There are now over 300 games in 48 states. The Coalition on Health and Fitness under the leadership of the International Health, Racquet and Sports Club Association, brings together organizations that promote legislation, deliver public service programs, and support Federal initiatives in the health and fitness areas.

Health Professionals

This is a particularly challenging area and one that has received attention in the United States Public Health Service, especially since President Dwight Eisenhower's 1955 heart attack motivated his physician, Paul Dudley White, to take action. At this Third International Conference on Nutrition and Fitness, Birrer [1] has described eloquently what we need to do. A number of projects are underway. For example, an NIH's NHLBI-funded program, Assisting Primary Care Providers with Lipid-Lowering Intervention (APPLI), is evaluating practical approaches and effectiveness of diet counseling in the clinical setting. Another, which is intended to be a template for patient physical activity counseling, is the CDC's Project PACE (Physician-based Assessment and Counseling for Exercise). PACE targets known, modifiable determinants of physical activity including self-efficacy, perceived barriers, and social support. The Public Health Service-initiated campaign to 'Put Prevention into Practice' provides a means to improve delivery of clinical preventive services, including nutrition assessment and dietary and physical activity counseling. This program would increase patient and provider education and improve the organization of these services in primary care provider offices and clinics.

Introducing the Physician's Rx: Exercise is a recent development from the President's Council on Physical Fitness and Sports.

Food Service and Healthy Food Choices

The scientific consensus on the relationship of diet to disease has compelled more attention to the kind of food that is provided to people in public programs like congregate and home delivered meals for the elderly, supplemental food and food vouchers for the poor, and school breakfast and lunch programs. Perhaps the most far-reaching is the USDA's initiative to bring its school meals programs into line with the *Dietary Guidelines for Americans* [2]. On a smaller scale, but no less critical, meals of the HHS Administration on aging programs are also required to be consistent with the *Dietary Guidelines for Americans.*

Nutrition Labeling

In the 1990s the United States Congress enacted legislation that required an overhaul of the food label on packaged foods. In response, FDA, in collaboration with the FSIS developed regulations for nutrition labeling of essentially all packaged foods. The new Nutrition Facts label, appearing on nearly all food products in 1994, has transformed the label's utility to guide healthy food choices by consumers and is stimulating a new health awareness by food manufacturers, as witnessed, for example by the plethora of nonfat, low fat, and reduced fat products appearing on supermarket shelves.

Food Safety

Safe and adequate food supplies are essential for proper nutrition. In the US, the HHS Food and Drug Administration (FDA) and the USDA Food Safety and Inspection Service (FSIS) bear primary responsibility for monitoring and assuring a safe food supply. Despite advances in technology, food-borne diseases continue to be a significant public health problem and require constant vigilance. Chemical substances also occur in food due to environmental contamination. Both present nutrition challenges [3]. One would expect that as the global markets increase and food produced on the other side of the world yesterday appears on American tables today, issues related to contamination may increase and will need to be addressed. New and more sustainable means of production may also be required to prevent such contamination.

Research and Surveillance on Diet, Physical Activity, and Health

Generation of new knowledge from research is the key to success in implementation efforts. Nearly half a billion dollars is spent annually across the Federal government on nutrition-related research, including research on public education and information [Interagency Committee on Human Nutrition Research, unpubl.]. This investment has been reflected in the leadership shown by our research institutions who long ago recognized the value of both sound nutrition and a physically active lifestyle. The landmark Framingham study of cardiovascular disease risk factors is still yielding information. A substantial amount of current knowledge about community-based prevention strategies has been learned from three U.S. research field trials for community-based health promotion – including diet and physical activity – to reduce cardiovascular disease. These three trials, funded by the NHLBI, are the Minnesota Heart Health Program, the Pawtucket Heart Health Program, and the Stanford Five-City Project. Recently, the government-wide Interagency Committee on Human Nutrition Research identified research on how to stimulate healthy food, nutrition, and physical activity behaviors, both individually and collectively, as one of three themes for priority focus, underscoring the continuing recognition of the critical nature of this endeavor.

Finally, we want to underscore the importance of data systems to assess and track progress. In this regard, the surveys and surveillance systems of the government-wide National Nutrition Monitoring and Related Research Program [4] provide the underpinning for policies and program directions for chronic disease reduction through provision of data and information on health and nutritional assessment, food consumption, attitudes and behaviors related to health, including physical activity practices, and the US food supply. Without this critical information, our efforts would be severely hampered and less effective.

Conclusion

In summary, there is a growing realization of the essential nature of sound nutrition and physical activity and that they go hand in hand. Public policy recognizes the importance of a collaborative approach to advancing healthful diet and physical activities patterns for young and old alike. We have made a number of advances in the dietary arena, but we still have a long way to go. We are on the brink of accelerated progress in the physical activity arena. The challenge is clear. Future public policies must emphasize the essential relationship between nutrition and physical activity and the potential alliances that will allow individual Americans to adopt healthy lifestyles. With the momentum of the 1996 Olympiad in the United States, we are ready to collectively accelerate progress to improve health prospects through healthful dietary practices and increased physical activity.

References

1   Birrer R: Physical activity in the prevention and management of cardiovascular disease. Third International Conference on Nutrition and Fitness, Athens, May 24–27, 1996. World Rev Nutr Diet. Basel, Karger, 1997, vol 82, pp 191–209.
2   US Department of Agriculture and US Department of Health and Human Services: Nutrition and Your Health: The Dietary Guidelines for Americans. Washington, USGPO, 1995.
3   United States Department of Agriculture, United States Department of Health and Human Services, United States Agency for International Development: Nutrition Action Themes for the United States: A Report in Response to the International Conference on Nutrition. Washington, USGPO, in press.
4   Wright J (ed): Interagency Board for Nutrition Monitoring and Related Research. Nutrition Monitoring in the United States: The Directory of Federal and State Nutrition Monitoring Activities. Hyattsville, Public Health Service, 1992.

Philip R. Lee, 200 Independence Avenue, S.W., Suite 716-G, Washington, DC 20201 (USA)

Simopoulos AP (ed): Nutrition and Fitness: Evolutionary Aspects, Children's Health,
Programs and Policies. World Rev Nutr Diet. Basel, Karger, 1997, vol 81, pp 114–121

....

National Policies Promoting Better Nutrition, Physical Fitness and Sports for All in China

Ji Di Chen

Research Division of Sports Nutrition and Biochemistry,
Institute of Sports Medicine, Beijing Medical University, Beijing, China

The Chinese government has always faced a great challenge to meet its people's need for food because of the huge population and a very limited arable land. The implementation of reform and open policies has been successful to bring about economic development, increase agricultural production, and increase the food supply, etc. For example, grain output was 435.29 million tons (383.5 kg/capita/year) in 1991, while it was 239.96 and 320.56 million tons in 1970 and 1980, respectively. The production of edible oil, meat, and fruit in 1991 was two to five times more than that of 1970 and 1980, and thus led to a remarkable improvement of the population's quality of life and health in recent years [1–3].

In connection with the increased food production, food consumption of Chinese people significantly increased as well in the past 40 years (table 1) [1, 3]. The updated nutrition survey in 1992 showed that the average energy intake of Chinese people has remained at 2,600 kcal (10,884 kJ) since 1986, but protein and fat intakes have increased continuously, especially for rural populations (table 2). The percentage of Body Mass Index (BMI) of <18.5 was reduced, and that of $BMI > 25$ increased, in Chinese adults 20–45 years of age (table 3) [1–3]. However, a small proportion of rural and mountain area populations are still facing nutritional deficiency problems, and some important policies to improve the nutritional status and fitness of people require attention [1, 3–5].

Table 1. The major food consumption of Chinese people between 1978 and 1992 (kg/capita/year)

Year	Grains	Vegetable oil	Meat	Poultry	Eggs	Aquatic products	Sugar	Wine
1978	196	1.60	8.42	0.44	1.97	3.50	3.42	2.57
1982	225	3.53	12.78	1.02	2.52	3.85	4.41	5.24
1986	253	5.17	15.53	1.72	5.20	5.33	6.04	8.97
1992	236	6.29	20.27	2.31	7.75	7.29	5.42	12.94

Data from 1993 Statistics Year Book of China.

Table 2. Dietary intake of energy, protein and fat of Chinese People between 1978 and 1992 (per capita/day)

Year	Energy kcal	Protein		Fat	
		g	% of total kcal	g	% of total kcal
1978	1,833	46.5	10.1	28.2	13.8
1982	2,271	54.7	9.6	41.4	16.4
1986	2,621	62.9	9.6	52.3	18.0
1992	2,597	62.2	9.6	61.4	21.3

Data from 1993 Statistics Year Book of China.

Improvement of Nutrition and Physical Fitness of People Should Be Taken Care of from Childhood

Children are the future of the world, and they are the most sensitive population in response to nutritional insufficiencies. Nutritional deficiencies are the most serious and commonly seen in children; henceforth, the growth and development level of children has been used to understand the nutritional status of the population. Although the trend of growth and development of Chinese children in the past 5 years has shown that the incidence of low weight decreased in most of the provinces, the decrease was less in rural areas as compared with cities. The incidence of low weight of <6-month-old children was 2.2% (city) and 6.9% (rural areas), respectively; and was 7.1% (city) and 23.1% (rural areas), respectively, of children 6–12 months in China. It has

Table 3. BMI of Chinese adults aged 20–45 years between 1982 and 1992

Areas	Years	BMI < 18.5	BMI > 25.0
City	1982	11.5	7.2
	1989	10.1	12.0
	1992	9.0	14.9
Rural	1982	9.0	5.5
	1989	7.7	7.5
	1992	8.0	8.4

Data from Chen, Chinese Academy of Preventive Medicine [1].

Table 4. The incidence of growth retardation rate of children of <5 years of age in urban and rural areas of China in 1992 (%)

Areas	Boys	Girls
Urban	11.4	11.5
Rural	39.3	40.5

Data from Chen [1].

been shown that the incidence of growth retardation of children in rural areas was more than three times greater as compared with that of the data in cities (table 4) [1].

Statistical analysis of the multifactors causing growth retardation of 132,923 children of less than 5 years of age showed that the main factors were: poverty, unsanitary conditions leading to drinking water contamination, diarrhea, lack of breast-feeding, low cultural level of parents, low income/person, lack of care for children, and sexual discrimination. Recent research confirmed that malnutrition holds an important position in the cause of death of children. About 55% of the diseased children had malnutrition, yet 80% of the malnutrition was of mild and medium degree. Malnutrition is an important factor undermining the health of children [1]. Although malnutrition of Chinese children under 5 years of age in cities is close to being solved, and the problems left are to promote breast-feeding and prevent overnutrition or nutrition imbalance, in rural and mountain areas malnutrition is still a prevalent problem. The period from 6 to 18 months is the

Table 5. Comparison of the incidence of diarrhea and respiratory disease in children of 6 months to 2 years of age with or without vitamin A supplement in 1990–1992 (person time/year)

Subjects	Diarrhea	Respiratory disease
With vitamin A supplement	0.76	0.52
With no vitamin A supplement	1.76	1.77
Reduction rate, %	57	71

Data from Chen [1].

most important period for children because the nutritional status of this period directly influences the growth and development thereafter until 5 years of age. Thus, to improve the nutritional status of children for better health, emphasis should be put on rural areas with the focal point of poverty alleviation.

Among the countermeasures to improve the nutritional status of the Chinese people, promotion of breast-feeding combined with poverty alleviation, especially in rural areas, is essential. An investigation showed that the total breast-feeding rate in rural areas of China has reached 92.4%, but the rates are still low in several provinces such as Sichuan, He-long-Jiang, and Fu-Jian. The attributable degree of risk for malnutrition in the areas of low breast-feeding ranged from 29 to 53% which indicated that carrying out breast-feeding may reduce 1/3 of the malnutrition of children under 5 years of age, and the course of disease could be shortened to about 1/3 of the original as well [1]. The effect of vitamin A supplementation in the reduction in the incidence of diarrhea and respiratory disease of children is significant. Results of vitamin A supplementation of 6-month- to 2-year-old children at three villages in the He-Bei Province showed that vitamin A intervention is a valuable health tool to reduce diarrhea and respiratory disease (table 5) [1].

'Soybean Action' is an ongoing plan, and developing soybean production has been suggested to be included in the national policy. Data showed that incidence of anemia in children was reduced by 17–24% in districts where soybean production increased 3.2 times. Soybean is a very good source of high-quality protein containing 40% protein with a good essential amino acid composition, which may also be beneficial to improve growth and development [1, 4].

Table 6. Comparison of the incidence of some major chronic diseases (%) in populations of >20 years of age from 9 provinces in 1992 with that of the data in 1986

Time and place	Hypertension	Coronary heart disease	Cerebral vascular disease	Chronic bronchitis
1986	48.90	16.01	7.00	34.56
1992				
Beijing	99.96	80.13	20.23	46.14
He-Bei	62.92	42.66	17.86	35.72
He-Luong-Jiang	55.70	53.30	20.89	71.11
Zhe-jiang	60.22	41.57	7.78	56.72
Guang-dong	40.96	145.47	13.00	37.04
Si-Chuan	48.56	22.45	16.84	106.63
Ning-xia	30.74	26.22	5.42	49.73

Data from Chen [1].

Educate and Guide Food Consumption Behavior and Develop Rational Markets

Food consumpton behavior of the Chinese people has changed simultaneously with progress in economic development. Consumption of, and demands for animal foods are continuously increasing, e.g. meat consumption has increased to 31–87 kg/capita/year for the top 10% income citizens, while it was 15–18 kg/capita/year for people of rural areas. At the same time the proportion of dietary energy from grains has been decreasing, year by year. These changes in food consumption are closely related to the increase of the incidence of chronic disease [6]. Comparison of the incidence of some major chronic diseases between 1986 and 1992 showed that the incidence of hypertension has increased onefold; cerebral vascular disease, twofold; and coronary heart disease, fourfold. In addition, the prevalence of overweight (BMI > 25) increased proportionately and reached 14.9% in people of 20–45 years of age in 1992 (table 6) [1]. Education of people to make use of traditional foods (mostly natural plants and fruits) which are beneficial to health, and controlling the overconsumption of animal and high-fat foods have become important strategies in pursuing healthy food consumption and dietary patterns, for people in cities. Prevention of nutritional imbalance is a task of top priority. A food consumption goal for the year 2000 has been formulated and published by the Chinese Nutrition Society [7]. The amount of food and nutrient intakes were carefully designed according to food production and food habits of the Chinese population, and were based on established nutritional principles. The food consumption goal provides a daily energy intake of about 10,000 kJ (2,400 kcal), of which 60% should be derived from cereals, 25–30% from fat, and 10–15% from protein (which includes animal protein and legumes).

The Chinese Government Will Pursue the 'Sports for All' Plan, Carry Out Physical Training Standards, and Monitor People's Physiques

In order to develop mass sports activities more extensively and improve people's physiques, the Chinese government has developed the 'Sports for All' plan and put it into the 2nd Chapter, 11th Item of the Sports Law of The People's Republic of China. At the same time, China will carry out the 'Instructor's Technical and Social Estate System for Social Physical Culture'. Sports instructors are responsible for guiding social-physical activities [8].

The 'Sports for All' plan was formulated under the conditions that: (1) Mass sports have been developed vigorously. (2) The health status of people has been greatly improved. (3) The effects of exercise activities in improving the people's total quality (including intellectually and physically) are significant and confirmed. (4) The awareness that 'exercise improves health status' needs to be strengthened, since sports facilities, management and related laws and regulations have not been perfected, and problems need to be solved step by step.

The 'Sports for All' plan has been published and has already been in action since October 1, 1995. The target of this plan up to the year 2010 is 'Work hard to achieve the well-coordinated development of sports, national economy, and social affairs; comprehensively improve the Chinese national physique and health level; and complete a basic "Sports for All" system provided with distinctive Chinese features'.

The significance of exercise activity for fitness lies in that it may change risk factors of chronic diseases, improve functional status, and improve psychological status and the capacity of coping with stress. The importance of exercise for fitness is becoming more prominent day by day [9]. 'Sports for All' has become a systematic plan of engineering with the target to improve people's health and fitness level. The focal point is on the youth of the population (including children and adolescents). The plan includes education of students to be conscious to establish a lifetime habit of exercise. Exercise for minorities, women, the elderly, and disabled will also be given great importance. Facilities and space for exercise will be expanded.

There have been a series of countermeasures including that the 'Sports for All' plan will be put into the overall program of the nation's economy and social development. The government will offer more effective leadership, management, and overall planning, etc. Among the measures, simple and convenient exercise and sports to fit different ages, sex, professions, and physical conditions will be popularized. A valuable legacy will be further developed of traditional Chinese sports, medical treatment, health care, rehabilitation, and the nation's traditional and recreational exercise.

Conclusion

The successful implementation of Chinese reform and open policies has brought about the increase of agricultural production, and thus led to significant improvements of its population's nutritional status and health in recent years. However, a small portion of rural and mountain area populations are still facing nutritional deficiency problems, and another portion of city populations are facing nutrition excess and/or imbalance problems. Therefore, some important policies worth attention to improve the nutritional status and fitness of people are as follows:
(1) Improvement of nutrition and physical fitness of people beginning in childhood.
(2) Promotion of breast-feeding combined with poverty alleviation in rural areas.
(3) Education and guidance of people's food consumption behavior and development of rational markets.
(4) Achievement of a well-coordinated development of sports, the national economy, and social affairs; comprehensive improvement of the Chinese national physique and health level; and completion of a basic 'Sports for All' system provided with distinctive Chinese features.

References

1   Chen CM: Report on the improving countermeasures of food and nutritional status in China during the year of 1990 to 1992. Chinese Academy of Preventive Medicine and State Statistics Bureau, 1995, pp 1–15.
2   Chen CM: Dietary guidelines for food and agriculture planning in China. The Compilation of International Symposium on Food, Nutrition and Social Economics Development. Beijing, China Sci Tech Press, 1991, pp 34–48.
3   Ge KY, Zhai FY, Yan HC, Chen L, Wang Q, Jia FM: The dietary and nutritional status of Chinese population in 1990. Acta Nutr Sin 1995;17:123–134.
4   Ge KY, Shen TF: Perfecting food policies and improving people's health. Acta Nutr Sin 1991;13: 376–380.

5   Child Nutrition Surveillance Working Team: The nutritional status of the pre-school children in some poor areas in China. The Compilation of International Symposium on Food, Nutrition, and Social Economics Development. Beijing, China Sci Tech Press, 1991, pp 64–69.

6   Zhao FJ: Studies on the relationship between dietary composition, health and disease. The Compilation of International Symposium on Food, Nutrition, and Social Economics Development. Beijing, China Sci Tech Press, 1991, pp 86–91.

7   Chinese Nutrition Society: The dietary guidance of the Chinese. Acta Nutr Sin 1990;12:1–10.

8   Department of Policy and Law and Regulations of China Sports Committee: Social Sports; in Department of Education, Science, and Culture of the Bureau of Legal System of The State Council (ed): Sports Law of Peoples Republic of China. Xin-Hua Publishing House, 1995, pp 3–4.

9   Chen JD: Benefits of physical activity; in Institute of Nutrition and Food Hygiene, Chinese Academy of Preventive Medicine (ed): International Symposium on Nutrition and Fitness, Symposium Proceedings. Institute of Nutrition and Food Hygiene, Chinese Academy of Preventive Medicine, 1994, pp 157–163.

Ji Di Chen, Research Division of Sports Nutrition and Biochemistry,
Institute of Sports Medicine, Beijing Medical University, 49 North Garden Road,
Hai Dian District, Beijing 100083 (China)

Simopoulos AP (ed): Nutrition and Fitness: Evolutionary Aspects, Children's Health,
Programs and Policies. World Rev Nutr Diet. Basel, Karger, 1997, vol 81, pp 122–127

....

National Programs and Policies Promoting Better Nutrition, Physical Fitness and Sports for All: Experiences from Africa

Catherine Siandwazi

Food and Nutrition Programme, Commonwealth Regional Health Community
Secretariat, for East, Central and Southern Africa, Arusha, Tanzania

African governments in close collaboration with the International Community have reemphasized their commitments to the goals of adequate nutrition for all. Common commitments were made at the World Summit for Children (1990), at the Conference on Hidden Hunger (1991), at the Organization of African Unity (OAU) Meeting on the African Child (1990), and various other African health ministers conferences. In addition, between 1992 and 1994, health ministers conferences adopted the theme 'The Food and Nutrition situation: collaborative efforts in ECSA' which helped in harnessing the political commitment developed at the global meetings for better resource allocation for nutrition in member countries [1–3].

Food and nutrition policies, plans of actions, and nutrition strategies have been developed at various levels by African governments with the intention of providing adequate nutrition for all different population groups. A major objective of all these is to enable the different population groups to produce and use food to meet their nutritional requirements.

In addition to these efforts aimed at improving nutrition for all, governments have developed the following:

(1) Guidelines on the relationship between diet and health based on extensive international scientific review.

(2) Dietary guidance to reflect a growing concern on prevention of diet-related noncommunicable diseases.

(3) Food goals which often express the need for certain foods or groups of foods to be consumed in a daily diet.

(4) Food and nutrition labelling for the purpose of assisting in selecting a healthy diet.

(5) Nutrition education packages which play a key role in promoting healthy diets and lifestyles.

(6) Departments within appropriate government ministries for sports development.

Monitoring national policies to promote nutrition in sports remains to be a major challenge for most African governments and institutions because the focus of most nutrition programs has been, and continues to be, in areas of preventing malnutrition, especially in children and women.

African governments need to be sensitized and stimulated to deliberately develop mechanisms to promote 'Nutrition in Sports' within the framework of national nutrition policies and beyond the present general focus.

Problem Definition

The CRHCS/ECSA region reiterates that the areas for high priority action remain protein energy malnutrition (PEM), micronutrient deficiencies and diet-related noncommunicable diseases.

When ECSA Food and Nutrition Cooperation was founded by the ministers of health in the region during the 1970s, PEM was the major problem facing the region. Although much work has been done in this area since then, the region still experiences high levels of malnutrition resulting from poverty, frequent drought periods, declining social sector spending, and the economic decline that characterized the region during the last decade. The situation of food and nutrition in the region has shown a steady decline, with droughts, food shortages, high rates of maternal and child malnutrition, vitamin A deficiency, nutritional anemia, and iodine deficiency disorders.[1] A recent review of the food and nutrition situation in the region indicated that: (1) The prevalence of malnutrition is on the increase. (2) Stunting rates are high, affecting about one-third of young children in ECSA. (3) Over 40% of women suffer from iron deficiency and other forms of malnutrition, leading to high maternal

[1] Brief description from the 'East Central and Southern Africa Food and Nutrition Strategy' prepared by the CRHCS for ECSA, January 1996; and summarizing an earlier paper ('The food and nutrition situation in ECSA: collaborative efforts in ECSA') prepared by C. Siandwazi and S. Hansch, Arusha, Tanzania, with technical assistance from the USAID funded Support for Analysis and Research in Africa (SARA) project, November, 1993.

mortality and low birth weights for children born to these mothers. (4) Diet-related noncommunicable diseases are becoming a major health problem. (5) The decline in production and consumption of indigenous foods is leading to household food insecurity.

Development and Implementation of the Framework for National Policies in Member Countries

In recognition of the role that food and nutrition interventions play in improving the health status in the region, the Health Ministers Conference of 1978 recommended the establishment of nutrition units in various government ministries. Directors and heads of nutrition institutions in the region met in 1979 and again in 1984, when the ECSA Food and Nutrition Co-operation (ECSAFAN) was formed under the name of Expert Committee on Food and Nutrition of the Health Ministers Conference.

The Commonwealth Regional Health Community Secretariat in the East, Central and Southern Africa region is spearheading efforts to integrate nutrition issues into strategies for sustainable development. Member governments have given support to the various strategies and interventions being developed to tackle problems of malnutrition and hunger in the region.

Protein energy malnutrition and micronutrient deficiencies (iodine, vitamin A, and iron) and dietary related noncommunicable diseases have been identified as the leading nutrition problems in the region, and many programs to tackle both the symptoms and causes have been developed, and are under implementation. Salt iodization, distribution of iron tablets and vitamin capsules, mounting of child feeding programs, and promotion of nutrition health education have all been done.

In recognition of the complex interplay between malnutrition, poverty, and development, the regional food and nutrition program is involved in a number of activities aimed at increasing the capacity of several sectors to tackle problems of food and nutrition. Some of these activities are: (1) Engaging in capacity building through training, research and advocacy to build on national and international political commitment to food and nutrition. (2) Promotion of program-driven training and research for cadres involved in food and nutrition programs. (3) Mobilization of indigenous resources (human and material) for improved nutrition in the region. (4) Establishing and strengthening of nutrition units in a number of government ministries in the region. (5) Promoting collaboration between Government, Non-Governmental, and International Development agencies in the formulation and implementation of food and nutrition programs.

An assessment of training and research capacities in the region has been undertaken within this context of exploring what resources the region has to tackle food and nutrition programs. It is expected that the results of this assessment will contribute to the better definition of strategies to tackle problems of food and nutrition in the region. In particular, action is expected to be taken in such areas as: (a) program management; (b) training and human resource development; (c) research; (d) production and utilization of indigenous plant and animal foods; (e) policy development and analysis; (f) advocacy; (g) change and its impact on nutrition.

Achievements Due to Implementation of the Framework for National Policies in Member Countries

Raising Regional Awareness in Food and Nutrition Issues, 1977–1984
It was in the latter half of the 1970s that health ministers in the region recognized the need to have a focal point for food and nutrition activities in each of the Ministries of Health. This decision was in response to the prevailing problem in protein energy malnutrition. The main achievements from this phase were: (1) Clearer articulation of food and nutrition problems. (2) Setting up of nutrition units in Ministries of Health. (3) Deployment of nutrition personnel in the health and agricultural sectors. (4) Regional exchange of experiences between ministries. (5) Nutrition problems were firmly identified as priorities in the health sector.

Definition and Consolidation of Regional Plans, 1985–1991
In the period 1985–1991, the regional food and nutrition program was defined, and the work of nutrition focal points was consolidated in the various countries. The main achievements from this period were: (1) Assessments that showed that micronutrient deficiencies and diet-related chronic diseases were emerging as a high priority problems. (2) Internal structure of nutrition units was elaborated upon. (3) Programs were defined in training, maternal and child nutrition, and nutrition in agricultural extension. (4) A regional training program was defined based on countries' needs. (5) The need for a full-time coordinator for food and nutrition in the region was identified. (6) Policy formulation in food and nutrition was identified as high priority to tackle the multifaceted nature of the problems; and some countries started work on this area.

Programing ECSA Activities, 1992–1995
It was in 1992 that the regional food and nutrition program came of age, with the deployment of an ECSA Food and Nutrition Coordinator in Arusha.

The main achievements from this period are: (1) A regional program started to take shape both in the countries and at the regional level. (2) Food and nutrition strategies developed in the region became better integrated into the international food and nutrition agenda at the ICN and National Plan of Action (NPA) for Women and Children. (3) Drought became a major development issue in the region. (4) Food and nutrition activities became affected by resource constraints brought about by economic reform programs in most of the countries. (5) Food and nutrition issues became part of the political agenda as ministers of health, agriculture, and economic planning became more active in addressing national and household food security issues. (6) There was increased commitment to food and nutrition programs in the region. (7) Food and nutrition policy work in the region continued and became intensified.

Intensifying Implementation of Activities, 1996–2000

In the coming 5-year period, the regional program intends to embark on a capacity building for national institutions so that they can better program food and nutrition activities into overall national development in each country. The main goals are to: (1) Support each national nutrition unit to prepare implementation programs. (2) Utilize existing institutional memory in the setting of priorities in the region. (3) Foster commitment to regional food and nutrition programs in all the countries. (4) Rigorously evaluate the relevance and role of ECSA Food and Nutrition Coordination to national programs. (5) Improve communications between countries, and with the ECSA Food and Nutrition Coordinator. (6) Mobilize more resources from national governments and donors for food and nutrition activities in each country, and to improve coordination. (7) Develop capacity for a regional network of experts in food and nutrition. (8) Support efforts of countries in the formulation of food and nutrition policies in the context of political, economic and social developments throughout the region.

Future Challenges

Monitoring national policies to promote nutrition in sports remains to be a major challenge for most African governments and Institutions because the focus of most nutrition programs has been, and continues to be, in areas of preventing malnutrition especially in children and women.

African governments need to be sensitized and stimulated to deliberately develop mechanisms to promote 'Nutrition in Sports' within the framework of national nutrition policies and beyond the present general focus.

References

1   Lenneiye NM, Siandwazi C, Tagwireyi JT: Training and Research Needs Assessment for Food and
     Nutrition Programmes, March 1996.
2   Siandwazi C: The East, Central and Southern Africa Food and Nutrition Strategy, December, 1995.
3   Siandwazi C, Hansch S: The Food and Nutrition situation in ECSA: Collaborative Efforts in ECSA,
     November, 1993.

Catherine Siandwazi, Coordinator, Food and Nutrition Programme, Commonwealth Regional
Health Community Secretariat, P.O. Box 1009, Arusha, Tanzania

Simopoulos AP (ed): Nutrition and Fitness: Evolutionary Aspects, Children's Health,
Programs and Policies. World Rev Nutr Diet. Basel, Karger, 1997, vol 81, pp 128–135

....

National Programs and Policies Promoting Better Nutrition, Fitness and Sports for All in Greece

Antonia-Leda Matalas

Department of Nutrition and Dietetics, Harokopio University, Athens, Greece

Sports in Greece: The Classical Heritage

The beneficial role of optimum physical fitness to areas other than military preparation was first postulated in classical Greece. In ancient Greek cities, all citizens were involved with regular exercise and participated in athletic competitions. Not only boys and men, but in several instances, girls as well, were trained in athletics from early childhood. Participation in sports was viewed as an obligation in an effort to develop one's mental and physical abilities in a proportionate manner, to become an able member of the society, good parent and companion.

The modern Greek state, founded in the 19th century, soon turned to the doctrines of the classical times. It is not a coincidence that, around the time when the revival of Olympic Games was realized, the Greek government proceeded to establish important legislation aiming at the improvement of physical fitness of all Greek citizens. In 1899, physical education was introduced to Greek schools 'in all degrees of education and for both genders, as a mandatory course and of prime importance' [1]. To facilitate the instructors' work, a detailed syllabus for physical education was prepared. The syllabus emphasized the military component of gymnastics; the so-called orthosomatic exercises, and various military-type exercises prevailed. Shooting was introduced as a sport in high schools; it was offered to boys only. Track and swimming also appeared in this curriculum, as well as rowing, the latter being addressed to boys only. At the same time, other legislative actions were taken by the government of Theotokis, such as the establishment of several local and national athletic competitions, the enactment of state sponsorship for all

Table 1. Physical education in primary and secondary schools: time planning [from refs. 3, 4]

	Primary school		High school	
	h/year (average)	% total time	h/year (average)	% total time
Gymnastics-physical skills	26	48	7	10
Sports	18	33	36	52
Track and field	6	11	21	29
Folk-dancing	4	7	7	10
Total	54		71	

athletic unions in the country, and the reorganization of the Gymnastics Academy, the school that trained instructors for physical education [1]. The Greek government proceeded to implement these policies simply following the trends that were born in Western Europe during the Enlightenment period and served the new social role of the modern state.

Current Policies Promoting Fitness for All in Greece

In the 20th century, physical education in Greece is approached from a different viewpoint and its role in health promotion is being appreciated [2]. As a result of this new approach, the rigid curriculum followed in the beginning of the century is enriched with an appreciable amount of outdoor activities and sports. The current curriculum incorporates performance of gymnastics, training in track and field, as well as sports, and instruction of Greek folk dances [3, 4]. In primary school, two hourly sessions of physical education are offered weekly throughout the academic year. Topics taught are shown in table 1 and include gymnastics-kinesiology (representing 41% of total instruction time), sports (representing 33% of total instruction time), training in track and field (representing 11% of total instruction time), and folk dancing (representing 7% of total time). In secondary school, three hourly sessions of physical education are offered weekly throughout the first and second years of the curriculum, and two-hourly sessions weekly during the remaining 4 years in secondary school. Instruction topics include sports, namely basketball, volleyball, football and handball (representing 51% of total instruction time), track and field (representing 29% of total instruction time), gymnastics (representing 10% of total instruction time), and folk-dancing (representing

10% of total instruction time). Attendance of the course is mandatory for all students.

Programs and ideas for the physical education curriculum at schools are developed by the Ministry of Education. Training of the student in athletics and sports is viewed as serving three major educational goals: maintenance of health, preservation of national culture, and social-moral strengthening of the student. As pointed out by Rontoyannis in his paper at this conference, in the core of physical education's scope as a course lies the development of motor-cognitive skills of the student. We know, however, that different types of physical activity are not equally efficient in preventing the development of degenerative conditions. This factor is not being taken into account in physical education programs of Greek schools and represents an area on which emphasis must be placed in the future, and research needs to be conducted.

In more recent decades the Greek government took additional policy measures aiming to promote fitness of the Greek population at large. In 1983, the movement of 'Sports for All', an international movement that was born within the European Community in the 1970s, found its legislative realization [5]. The movement's goal, as defined by its proponents, lies in the improvement of life quality through promotion of health and prevention of disease, development of better social life, and improvement of the citizen's relation to his natural environment. The first programs, at an experimental stage, were tried out in Greece, in 1982–1983. In 1985, the Office for the Development of Sports was founded, having as its main task to promote the 'Sports for All' movement [5]. The Office for the Development of Sports, a subdivision of the General Secretariat of Athletics in the Ministry of Culture, launched an unprecedented campaign to attract peoples' participation to new sports programs. By the late 1980s, a wide spectrum of programs had been developed and offered in most cities and towns of the country. Particular programs included summer programs for children, youth programs, programs for women, and programs for professionals. Specific programs have also been addressed to men in military service, to the elderly, to children with special needs, to persons recovering from addiction, and to prisoners [5, 6]. Participation in various programs reached 670,000 persons in 1987, a number that reflects 7% of the country's general population [5]. Participation dropped severely after 1991: in each of the two periods of 1993–94 and 1994–1995 only about 100,000 people were recruited into programs offered [Greek Ministry of Culture, unpubl. data]. Table 2 shows the particular programs that were implemented within the 'Sports for All' movement during the period 1991–1993. Programs for women have been particularly successful, as women participated at a rate that was 1.5 times higher than the one observed among men [Greek Ministry of Culture, unpbl. data].

Table 2. 'Sports for All' programs implemented by the Greek Ministry of Culture during the years 1991–1993

> Programs for children	> Programs for women
Sports and child	Sports and woman
Child and sea	
Child and mountain	> Programs for men in military servie
	Sports and army
> Programs for young people	> Programs for persons with special needs
Youth and dancing	Sports and third age
Youth and mountain	Sports and children with special needs
> Programs for professionals	Sports and addicts
Football and basketball	Sports in prison

Despite these governmental efforts, Greeks are less fit than they used to be in previous decades. This can be documented by the increasing rates of obesity observed among Greek men and women, while prevalence of obesity among Greek children, estimated at about 20%, is alarming [7]. One can speculate some reasons for these changes: everyday life in modern Greek urban centers involves minimal physical activity, in contradiction with the lifestyle that prevailed until the 1970s. At the same time, availability of public recreational centers in cities is scarce. Children are homebound and have no chance to engage in spontaneous physical activities as children in small towns and villages do. The vast majority of the Greek population lives in cities – 40% of the country's population live in the greater urban area of Athens. This is the result of the urbanization that occurred during the 1960s and 1970s. Designing programs for children is, there-fore, of vital priority, as the limited time allocated to physical activity by their school program cannot substitute for the lost play-time.

Greek Diet: The Classical Heritage

Moving from fitness and sports, to nutrition, I would like to briefly review some of the fragmentary data that exist on the diets followed by ancient Greek athletes. Diogenis Laeritus (3rd century AD) wrote that most ancient Greek athletes were trained on a diet of dry figs, moist cheese, and wheat, and that this pattern changed abruptly and focused on meat [8]. Pausanias (2nd century AD) attributed this change in the athletes' diet to Dromeus of Stymphalos, a long-distance runner who trained exclusively on meat, and won two consecutive victories in the Olympic games of 484 and 480 BC [9]. Epictetus (2nd century

Table 3. Seven-countries, study: mean percentage of energy intake from fat and 15-year death rates per 10,000 'healthy' men aged 40–59 years at entry, in selected cohorts [from ref. 11]

Cohort	Mean % of energy intake from			15-year death rate	
	Total fats	saturated fatty acids	monounsaturated fatty acids	all causes	CHD
Non-Mediterranean Europe					
East Finland	38.5	23.7	11.9	2,270	1,202
Zutphen, the Netherlands	38.0	20.2	12.5	1,825	636
Slavonia, Yugoslavia	31.9	13.6	13.3	2,365	389
Mediterranean Europe					
Crevalcore, Italy	27.0	8.9	11.4	2,046	424
Crete, Greece	36.1	7.7	25.8	855	38
Corfu, Greece	33.0	6.4	18.3	1,317	202

AD) wrote that Olympic victors avoided desserts and used wine sparingly [10]. Philostratus (3rd century AD) disapproved of the athletic diet in his era and noted that the diet of athletes had shifted to white bread sprinkled with poppy seeds, and intakes of both fish and pork [11].

The diet that was followed among Greeks in classical times was based on barley and wheat, olives and olive oil, onions and some other vegetables, figs, grapes and wine, fish and cheese [12, 13]. This pattern was carried over to the 19th century with only a few changes [14]. In the 19th century, new food items were introduced to the diet of the Greeks, such as tomatoes, potatoes, and green peppers. This pattern that was created by the end of the 19th century is what we call the traditional Greek diet. This traditional dietary pattern, as it has been documented among Greek islanders, has been put forward by many as a model of what a prudent diet should be. Diets followed by the Cretans in the 1960s were found to be associated with low incidence of ischemic heart disease and all-cause mortality rates, assertions that resulted initially from data collected as part of the Seven Countries Study [15, 16]. Some of these findings are shown in table 3. The dietary habits of Greeks have changed dramatically since then, as it was shown by investigations carried out by Kafatos and his collaborators in Crete. Consumption of saturated fat among Cretans in 1988 was found to be significantly higher compared to the consumption observed in the 1960s [17]. The abandonment of the traditional dietary pattern was mainly the result of the increased rates of urbanization that occurred in the country during the 1960s and 1970s. During the past three decades the Greeks quickly and easily adopted a westernized diet [18].

Changes in dietary intake are followed by changes in biochemical markers [19, 20] and increased rates of cardiovascular disease observed nationwide among men and women since the 1970s [21, 22]. These and other findings suggest that new dietary habits adopted by Greeks have detrimental effects to public health and precipitate increased rates of degenerative diseases. Research done by several laboratories worldwide on the biological role of some of the components of the Mediterranean-type diets, support this theory [23–27].

The ancient spirit was revived at the turn of the 20th century in athletics and sports; it seems that the turn of the 21st century is the right time for Greeks to rediscover their ancient dietary heritage. Similar to athletics and sports, nutrition carries a cultural as well as health component. The difference is that while the Olympics and the other big athletic events of antiquity were abolished soon after the advent of Christianity, dietary habits continued to evolve and were sustained throughout the centuries.

Nutrition Research and Policies in Greece

At the present time there are few centers in the country that have been working in educating the population on the benefits of the traditional dietary patterns, and which have conducted intervention studies. No combined effort, in the form of a national policy, however, was ever implemented in Greece, so that the basic characteristics of the traditional dietary pattern be maintained.

Unlike physical exercise, where the responsible governmental agencies are few (Ministries of Education and Culture), the situation in the area of nutrition is less well defined. This can be illustrated by considering the chaotic status that exists in the area of food safety and quality. The Ministry of Economics, the Ministry of Agriculture, the Ministry of Commerce, and the Police Department, are all involved in one way or another in screening the food supply for safety and quality, and regulating food production in the country – each one by being responsible for a different group of foods or food services. In Greece there is no agency equivalent to what the Food and Drug Administration (FDA) represents in the US.

During the past few years, the role of nutrition in promoting public health has begun to be appreciated by the Greek government. Now the time is ripe for nutrition, and the key role it plays in maintaining vitality and preventing disease, to be included in the new food, agricultural, health care, and education policies in the country. For example, in a new health-care system, identification of nutritional status problems can become a routine, and nutritional status should be as vital a sign of health as are blood pressure and pulse rate.

Nutrition as a scientific discipline has been developed by some higher educational institutions: The Athens School of Public Health, the Department of Medicine at the University of Crete, the Department of Food Technology and Nutrition at the Technological Educational Institutions in Thessaloniki, and the Department of Dietetics at Harokopio University in Athens. These schools, listed above according to the chronological order of their foundation, have developed courses on nutrition which have been included as valuable components of their study curricula. Intervention studies, as well as epidemiological studies, have also been conducted by these centers, often in collaboration with other European centers. In addition, an appreciable amount of work has been done on formulating food composition databases representative of the local food supply: such food tables are lacking at the moment. The Department of Social Medicine on Crete has pursued the Seven Countries Study and documented the changes in the dietary habits of the Cretans since the sixties, mentioned above. It has also been very active in designing and implementing nutrition intervention programs on the island of Crete. Target populations for such programs have been pregnant women, adolescents, children, as well as adults at high risk for cardiovascular disease. The Athens School of Public Health has undertaken food consumption surveillance projects, as well as large-scale epidemiological studies launched by the European Union.

The importance attributed to improving the nutritional status of all citizens by the Greek government, however, has been primarily demonstrated by the fact that the Greek government established a Department of Dietetics at the University level in 1990. The new Department of Dietetics, housed at Harokopio University, accepted its first students in 1994, and from now on will be training qualified dieticians. It is currently in the process of setting the base for its research directions and establishing links and collaborations with European and American centers in the field of nutrition. The Harokopio University aspires to bring nutrition and fitness-related research activities together. Because development of policy measures is needed to serve as a bridge between research and practice in the community, the new department will also strive to promote public policy-making in the areas of nutrition and fitness in Greece.

References

1   Greek Government: Themidos Code 1899. Themidos Law Library, No 13, 1899, p 81.
2   Greek Institute of Pedagogics. Physical Education: Guidelines for the Instructor, in press.
3   Greek Ministry of Education and Religion: Analytical Syllabus and Directions for the Instruction of Physical Education in Primary School. Athens, 1988.
4   Greek Ministry of Education and Religion: Analytical Programs for Physical Education in Gymanasium and Lyceum. Athens, 1990.

5   Nikitas N: Sports For All: Theoretical Framework. Athens, Telethrion, 1993, 2/e, pp 13–15, 117, 137.
6   Greek Ministry of Culture: The Administrative Framework for the 'Sports for All' Programs. Official Bull. Athens, 1995.
7   Kafatos A, Panagiotakopoulos G, Bastakis N, Trakas D, Stoikidou M, Pantelakis S: Cardiovascular risk factors status of Greek adolescents in Athens. Prevent Med 1981;10:173–186.
8   Diogenes Laertius: Lives of Eminent Philosophers (translated by Hicks RD). London, Heinemann, 1925.
9   Pausanias: Description of Greece (translated by Jones WHS). 5 vols. New York, Putnam, 1918–1935.
10   Epictetus: The Discourses of Epictetus; with Encheridion and Fragments (translated by Long G, Burt AL). New York, 1988.
11   Philostratus: Concerning Gymnastics (translated by Woody T). Ann Arbor, 1936.
12   Grivetti LE: Nutrition past-nutrition today: Prescientific origins of nutrition and dietetics. 2. Legacy of the Mediterranean. Nutr Today 1991;26:18–29.
13   Waterlow JC: Diet of the classical period of Greece and Rome. Eur J Clin Nutr 1989;43(suppl 2): 3–12.
14   Matalas A, Grivetti LE: Dietary assessment of 19th century Greek sailors: Analysis of the katastichon of the Konstantinos. Food Foodways 1994;5:353–389.
15   Keys A, Menotti A, Karnoven M, Aravanis C, Blackburn H, Buzina R, Djordjevic B, Dontas A, Fidanza F, Keys A, Kromhout D, Nredeljkovic S, Punsar S, Seccareccia F, Toshima H: The diet and 15-year death rate in the seven contries study. Am J Epidemiol 1986;124:903–915.
16   Keys A, Aravanis C, Van Buchem FSP, Blackburn H, Buzina R, Djordjevic B, Fidanza F, Karvonen M, Kimura N, Menotti A, Nedeljkovic S, Puddu V, Punsar S, Taylor H: The diet and all-causes death rate in the seven countries study. Lancet 1981;ii:58–61.
17   Kafatos A, Kouroumalis I, Vlachonikolis I, Theodorou C, Labadarios D: Coronary-heart-disease risk-factor status of the Cretan urban population in the 1980s. Am J Clin Nutr 1991;54:591–598.
18   Matalas A, Grivetti LE: Mediterranean diet in the 19th and 20th century: The case of two ship crews and their provisions. Int J Food Sci Nutr 1993;44:261–279.
19   Aravanis C, Mensik RP, Karalias N, Christodoulou B, Kafatos A, Katan M: Serum lipids, apolopoproteins and nutrient intake in rural Cretan boys consuming high-olive-oil diets. J Clin Epidemiol 1988;41:1117–1123.
20   Fordyce MK, Christakis G, Kafatos A, Duncan R, Cassidy J: Adipose tissue fatty acid composition of adolescents in a US–Greece cross-cultural study of coronary heart disease and risk factors. J Chron Dis 1993;36:481–486.
21   WHO: World Health Statistics Annual. Geneva, WHO Statistics Division, 1991, 1992, p 8.
22   WHO: World Health Statistics Annual. Geneva, WHO Statistics Division, 1988.
23   Grundy SM: Comparison of monounsaturated fatty acids and carbohydrates for lowering plasma cholesterol. N Engl J Med 1986;314:745–748.
24   Gurr MI, Nazeli B, Ganatra S: Dietary fats and plasma lipids. Nutr Res Rev 1989;2:63–86.
25   Mensik RP, Katan MB: Effects of monounsaturated fatty acids versus complex carbohydrates on HDL in healthy men and women. Lancet 1987;i:122–125.
26   Renaud S: From the cradle of our civilization the diet to effectively prevent CHD. Eur J Clin Nutr 1991;45(suppl 2):96–99.
27   Simopoulos AP: The Mediterranean food guide. Nutr Today 1995;30:54–61.

Antonia-Leda Matalas, Department of Nutrition and Dietetics, Harokopio University,
70 Venizelou Street, GR–17671 Kalithea, Athens (Greece)

Simopoulos AP (ed): Nutrition and Fitness: Evolutionary Aspects, Children's Health, Programs and Policies. World Rev Nutr Diet. Basel, Karger, 1997, vol 81, pp 136–147

....

National Policies for Promoting Physical Activity, Physical Fitness and Better Nutrition in Europe

Willem van Mechelen

Institute for Research in Extramural Medicine and Department of Social Medicine, Faculty of Medicine, Vrije Universiteit, Amsterdam, The Netherlands

The relation between physical activity, physical fitness and health can be described with a conceptual model presented by Bouchard (fig. 1) [1]. Based on current knowledge, it is generally accepted that both physical activity and physical fitness are independent markers of health status and functional independence. It is obvious that the mutual relations between physical activity, physical fitness and health status are influenced by a wide variety of 'other' factors, such as genetics, physical and social environment, and lifestyle factors, such as smoking, alcohol consumption, and nutrition.

From a nutritional point of view, it is noteworthy that low levels of physical activity and physical fitness are both associated with overweight. From that perspective, maintaining energy balance, i.e. the balance between energy intake and energy expenditure, is obviously of importance. There are, however, many other relations between nutrition, physical activity, physical fitness and health status, e.g. a high serum cholesterol is associated with low levels of physical activity, and a high energy intake from saturated fat.

Physical activity, physical fitness and nutrition are, in their mutual relation to health status, all modifiable by a change of lifestyle. Such a change of lifestyle will not only influence an individual's health status, but will also have a beneficial influence on the public health status of a nation. It is therefore interesting to know to what extent national policies exist that are aimed at promoting a physically active lifestyle, at enhancing levels of physical fitness and at promoting better nutrition.

The purpose of this paper is to give a brief overview of public policies that promote (1) a physically active lifestyle; (2) the enhancement of levels of

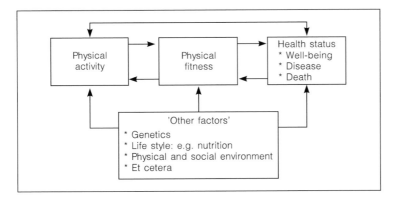

Fig. 1. Conceptual model describing the relations between physical activity, physical fitness, health status and 'other factors' (after Bouchard [1]).

physical fitness, and (3) better nutrition within Europe, either at a national or at a pan-European level.

Method of Obtaining Information

Given the fact that the purpose of this paper is to describe national and trans-European public policies based on governmental policy statements, statements of interest groups, etc., it is very difficult to obtain information from modern electronic retrieval systems, such as CD-ROM, MEDLINE®, etc. The political and social structure differs among countries and most official national documents are published in the so-called 'grey literature'. Consequently, the information presented here is predominantly gathered through a formal and informal network of experts. In this way, information was obtained about the promotion of physical activity, the prevention of sports injuries (as a negative health outcome of physical activity), the enhancement of levels of physical fitness and the promotion of better nutrition.

Promotion of a Physically Active Lifestyle

It is now widely accepted that a physically active lifestyle is associated with reduced cardiovascular mortality and all-cause mortality [2]. Also a wide variety of other disease states are associated with a physically inactive lifestyle, such as hypertension, non-insulin-dependent diabetes mellitus, osteoporosis, obesity and certain forms of cancer [2]. In addition, regular exercise is beneficial in the treatment of mild depression and anxiety [2]. When looking at the public health burden of a sedentary lifestyle, it was estimated by Powell and Blair [3] that in the US 35% of all coronary heart disease deaths, 32% of all colon cancer deaths, and 34% of all diabetes deaths could be attributed to a sedentary lifestyle. For obvious reasons, it thus makes sense to promote a physically active lifestyle.

Many initiatives throughout the world have been taken to promote a physically active lifestyle. For an overview, one is referred to Blair et al. [4]. Initiatives or statements at the European level will be briefly discussed below.

Two recommendations were made recently by the 'Committee of Ministers' of the member states of the Council of Europe, in which the significance of physical activity for society was stressed:

(1) In Recommendation No.R(95)16 on 'Young People and Sport', it was stated that young people should be able to participate in physical activities, both at school and during leisure time. In this recommendation concern was expressed that the time allotted to physical education or physical activities within the school system is often insufficient and that young people who are not involved in sport and physical activities have low levels of physical fitness [5]. The recommendation also contains a manifesto in which the member states are encouraged to set up programs among the youth that, 'ensure progression into a lifelong involvement in physical activity and sport' [5].

(2) In Recommendation No.R(95)17 on 'The Significance of Sport for Society', the Committee of Ministers of the member states of the Council of Europe note, 'the importance of sport in fostering good health and well-being in society'. Because of this they encourage people of all ages to take up regular moderate-to-vigorous physical exercise for at least half an hour daily as part of the daily activities. They also state that in stimulating a physically active lifestyle, priority should be given to finding and offering opportunities to sedentary and irregularly active people, and that the risk of sustaining a sports injury should be reduced [6].

More recently, in 1996, at the initiative of the European Commission (DG V; Employment, Industrial Relations and Social Affairs, and Public Health), a start was made with the establishment of a European network of experts involved in the 'Promotion of health-enhancing physical activity in the European Union member states'. The network is named 'Europe on the Move'. The purpose of this network is described as, 'to develop the rationale, approaches, principles and strategic guidelines of health-enhancing physical activities of the European countries'. At a first meeting of the network held in early 1996 representatives of 14 European countries made the following recommendations [7]: (1) development and adoption of public policy favoring health-enhancing physical activity; (2) creation of environments which facilitate health-enhan-

Table 1. Initiatives within Europe to promote a physically active lifestyle [7]

Country	National policy	Nationwide activities
Austria	–	national walking program
Belgium	–	youth sport campaign
Denmark	–	prevention ischemic heart disease
Finland	+	active population to be increased with 10% in the 40- to 60-year-old range
France	–	some programs with a narrow scope
Germany	–	no clear picture due to organization of health care system
Ireland	–	focal initiatives to increase participation in an active lifestyle
Italy	–	research and information-oriented programs on healthy habits in youth financed and organized by CONI
Netherlands	+	'Netherlands on the Move', target groups: elderly, children, working population, chronically ill
Spain (Catalonia)	±	advisory board that promotes physical activity
Sweden	–	national program in preparation, some local initiatives
United Kingdom	+	national program: promote regular physical activity

cing physical activity; (3) strengthening of community action which fosters health-enhancing physical activity; (4) facilitation of the development of personal resources for health-enhancing physical activity; (5) provision of services necessary for health-enhancing physical activity.

Next to the above-mentioned initiatives at a pan-European level, there are in some of the European countries initiatives to promote physical activity at a national level. A brief description of these initiatives is given below (see also table 1).

In Finland there has been a nationwide government endorsed action called 'Finland on the Move'. The purpose of this initiative was to organize local sports centers to promote increased physical activity by tailoring existing resources to local needs and conditions. The target group for this action included the entire Finnish population. The action specifically aimed at the support and stimulation of local initiatives to enhance a physically active lifestyle, through financial support, through training and consultation of those wanting to set up a local initiative, through facilitating communication between projects participating in 'Finland on the Move' and through the authorization of local initiative as being part of the nationwide program [4, 8]. In the United Kingdom there is a nationwide health-enhancing strategy named 'Strategy Statement on Physical Activity', which has been approved by the Minister of

Health. The aim of the strategy is to encourage increased participation in physical activity of a moderate intensity as part of everyday life. Like the US American College of Sports Medicine/Centers for Diseases Control (ACSM/CDC) recommendation [2], a minimum of 30 min of moderate physical activity on at least 5 days per week is advocated. This message is being promoted by national bodies such as the National Health Education Authority by mass media campaigns and the distribution of a newsletter entitled 'Let's Get Physical'. In the United Kingdom, the importance of a physically active lifestyle is also recognized by the Royal College of Physicians [4]. The Dutch government has recently explicitly stated in official documents the significance of inactivity as a risk factor for ill-health and has therefore made the promotion of a physically active lifestyle part of preventive strategies [9]. Consequently, in The Netherlands there is a national program to stimulate a physically active lifestyle. Taking the Finnish program as an example, it is called 'The Netherlands on the Move'. It is financed and endorsed by the Dutch government. Its main objective is to enlarge the proportion of the population which is physically active. 'The Netherlands on the Move' tries to reach its goals through improvement of knowledge and through promoting changes of the Dutch infrastructure. Currently, the program is aimed at two target groups: the elderly (55+) and the chronically ill. As in the United Kingdom, in The Netherlands the promotion of a physically active lifestyle is also endorsed and/or recognized by other important bodies, such as the Dutch Heart Foundation, and the National Institute of Public Health and the Environment [10].

According to the progress report of the first meeting of the European network 'Europe on the Move', there are no other nationwide government endorsed programs that promote a physically active life style. There are, however, quite a number more of focal initiatives going on (table 1) [7].

It should be noted that so far none of the initiatives mentioned in this section have been evaluated scientifically.

Prevention of Sports Injuries

In the seventies and eighties throughout Europe, the participation in sports activities was promoted, rather than promoting a broader physically active lifestyle. One of the unwanted side effects of participation in sports is the risk to sustain injuries. This was recognized by the Council of Europe, and a European project named 'Sports Injuries and Their Prevention' was launched. The project consisted of a series of expert seminars held between 1986 and 1988. Twelve European countries participated in the project, who committed themselves to reduce the incidence rate and severity of sports injuries by increasing knowledge, by conducting research, and by disseminating the study results. The seminars served as a platform to exchange and coordinate the scientific efforts made in the various member states. The project was carried out in two phases in each country: the problem was identified in the first phase; and prevention programs were implemented in the second phase. The program has led to substantial scientific output, for which one is referred to van Mechelen et al. [11] and van Vulpen [12]. In The Netherlands for instance, the program also led to a nationwide mass media campaign to reduce the number of sports injuries. Although this campaign, as such, was not evaluated scientific-ally, the results of two nationwide surveys, one carried out before the start of the campaign [13] and one carried out recently [14] suggest that the campaign has been successful in stabilizing the extent of the sports injury problem.

Enhancement of Levels of Physical Fitness

Again by the Council of Europe, considerable input was given to nationwide initiatives to enhance levels of physical fitness of the people living in these member states. This initiative is called EUROFIT. The initiative started off with EUROFIT for children and was later followed by EUROFIT for adults.

EUROFIT for Children
Following a number of expert seminars on the desirability of establishing a uniform battery to test the physical fitness of schoolchildren, the committee of the ministers of the Council of Europe adopted a recommendation (No.R(87)9) on 'The EUROFIT Tests of Physical Fitness' [15]. In this recom-mendation, a number of considerations were laid down as to why the measure-ment of physical fitness in children is important. Some of these considerations were, 'physical fitness is an important component, not only of sport and physical education, but also of health and health education, and is necessary for a state of well-being' and 'testing of physical fitness of children will provide important data to be used for the working out of national policies connected with children, health, nutrition, physical education and sport' [15]. The EURO-FIT for children test battery is made up of nine different tests, all measuring different dimensions and factors of physical fitness. Also, measurements of anthropometric data are included in the test battery (table 2).The test results can be evaluated either by comparing the results of the same individual over time, or by comparison with national reference tables. The dissemination of the test within Europe is acceptable (table 3) [16] and there are now national reference tables in 5 countries. The manual has also been translated into Hungarian and French. The test is also widely used in Northern Ireland.

Table 2. Dimensions and factors of physical fitness that constitute the EUROFIT for children test battery [15]

Dimension	Factor	EUROFIT for children test item
Cardiorespiratory endurance	cardiorespiratory endurance	20 m shuttle run test bicycle ergometer test (PWC$_{170}$)
Strength	static strength explosive strength (power)	handgrip standing broad jump
Muscular endurance	functional strength trunk strength	bent arm hang sit-ups
Speed	running speed speed of limb movement	10×5 m shuttle run plate tapping
Flexibility	flexibility	sit and reach
Balance	whole body balance	flamingo balance
Anthropometric measures		height weight skinfolds: % body fat

Table 3. Age- and sex-specific references of EUROFIT for children available in different European countries [16]

Country	Sex and age group
Italy	boys and girls 12–14 years
Spain (Catalonia)	boys and girls 13–18 years
Belgium	boys and girls 6–12 years boys and girls 13–18 years
Latvia	boys and girls 11–17 years
The Netherlands	boys and girls 12–16 years

EUROFIT for Adults

EUROFIT for adults is again an initiative of the Council of Europe. In order to establish EUROFIT for adults, the same procedure was followed as with EUROFIT for children. First there were two seminars at which experts decided on the content of the test battery, and then a handbook was produced by a smaller number of experts. The time frame in which the handbook for

Table 4. Dimensions, components and factors of health-related physical fitness that constitute the EUROFIT for adults test battery [17]

Dimension	Component	Factor	EUROFIT for adults test item
Aerobic fitness	maximal aerobic power	maximal aerobic power	2 km walk test, bicycle test or 20 m shuttle run test
Musculoskeletal fitness	muscle strength and muscle endurance	trunk muscle endurance leg muscle power arm muscle endurance hand muscle strength	dynamic sit up vertical jump bent arm hang hand grip
	flexibility	trunk flexion shoulder mobility	side bending or sit and reach shoulder abduction
Motor fitness	balance speed	whole body balance hand movement speed	single leg balance plate tapping
Anthropometric measures	height weight skinfolds waist girth/hip girth		Body Mass Index (weight for height) sum of skinfolds (estimate body fat) waist-hip ratio (estimate body fat distribution)

Physical activity and health questionnaire

adults was produced was much shorter than that for the children's handbook, because of the experience gained with EUROFIT for children. EUROFIT for adults differs from the EUROFIT for children in that it has a broader perspective, aiming not only at the measurement of physical fitness, but also at the measurement of physical activity and at health promotion. It primarily focusses on health-related fitness and not on performance-related fitness. It also addresses the issue of criterion-based references for fitness versus population-based references. Until now, EUROFIT for adults lacks formal approval by the member states and there are no population-based national references available. In the handbook for adults, the purposes of EUROFIT for adults are described as follows [17]:

(1) assessing the status of health-related fitness of individuals, communities, subpopulations and populations; (2) evaluating the levels of health-related fitness in relation to standard population norms and when possible to criterion values, and (3) providing a knowledge base and facilitating actions aimed at promoting health-related physical fitness and physical activity.

The target population for EUROFIT for adults is the healthy and functionally independent working age population from 18 to 65 years of age. The test items included in the EUROFIT for adults test battery are given in table 4. EUROFIT for adults also contains a recommendation with regard to health screening prior to participating in physical fitness testing. Finally, references are given in the handbook for most of the tests based on national surveys conducted in the United Kingdom (the Allied Dunbar Fitness Survey) and Sweden (the LIV90 survey).

Promotion of Better Nutrition

With regard to national policies promoting better nutrition, hardly any information could be obtained, with the exception of The Netherlands where, in 1987, the Dutch government has established a Steering Committee on Healthy Nutrition. This steering committee is a cooperative body composed of representatives of the Dutch government and of production, trade, information and consumer interest organizations in the field of food and nutrition. The objective of the steering committee is the implementation of the 'Guidelines for Healthy Nutrition' of The Netherlands Nutrition Council. After a preparation period in a mass media campaign from 1991 to 1995, the emphasis was placed on the reduction of fat intake with the slogan 'Keep fatty food intake in check'. The campaign first aimed at raising public awareness of the problem, then aimed at a change of attitude towards eating less fatty foods, and finally provided information on the taste and costs of a less fatty diet. This campaign showed effectiveness in terms of a shift of consumer habits towards the use of low-fat foods. However, it was also found that the public still are not able to make an adequate estimation of their own fat intake. Therefore, it was concluded that future campaigns should aim at increasing public awareness of the actual fat intake, and that the public should also be given support for behavioral change [Dutch Steering Committee on Healthy Nutrition, pers. commun.].

At the pan-European level, only some information regarding joint European research projects was found, as well as limited information regarding two disease-oriented health-promotion campaigns in which the importance of a healthy diet was put forward.

Examples of Joint Research Projects on Nutrition within Europe

The Seven Countries Study was initiated in 1960 in seven European countries. In this study, 16 different cohorts were measured with the aim to study risk factors for coronary heart disease. Data on the average food composition of each cohort are available and used in ecological studies on coronary heart disease, cancer and chronic obstructive pulmonary disease [10].

The European Prospective Investigation into Cancer and Health (EPIC) is a multicenter cohort study on cancer coordinated by the World Health Organization (WHO). Seven countries participate in this study: Germany, Greece, France, Italy, The Netherlands, Spain and the United Kingdom. The main objectives of this study are the quantification of cross-cultural dietary patterns in Mediterranean and northern European countries and testing hypotheses on diet, nutritional status and cancer incidences for the most common sites. The study started in 1993 and data collection will last until 1997 [10].

As part of the European Healthy Cities Project in 5 European cities – Eindhoven (Netherlands), Valencia (Spain), Liverpool (United Kingdom), Horsens (Denmark), and Rennes (France) – the efficacy of health education aimed at 'a healthy diet' was evaluated. The project started in 1990 and was conducted using supermarkets as a base for the dissemination of information. The project was recently evaluated [18]. One of the outcomes of the study was that increasing knowledge about a healthy diet, as such, does not improve dietary habits. Dietary habits are determined by a mixture of determinants that should all be taken into account when trying to change the public's nutritional habits, i.e. personal, social, cultural and environmental factors.

Disease-Oriented Health Education on Better Nutrition

In 1987, the European Commission started a program called 'Europe Against Cancer'. Both research and health education programs aimed at the reduction of cancer mortality were initiated as part of this program. In 1994 health educational efforts of the program focussed on the relation between nutrition and cancer [Dutch Cancer Society, pers. commun.].

The Heart Foundations of Europe cooperate in the 'European Heart Network'. This network recognizes the role of an unhealthy diet in a wide variety of diseases, such as cardiovascular disease, some forms of cancer, non-insulin-dependent diabetes mellitus, gastrointestinal and liver diseases, and dental caries. As part of their activities, the members of the network promote in their own countries healthy eating habits by providing information on and taking action with regard to items such as nutrition labelling, canteen menus, healthy cooking classes, healthy eating in the work place, nutrition and health claims, cholesterol consensus, the production of a 'light-hearted cookbook', supermarket involvement, etc. The network cooperates closely with the European Community [19].

Concluding Remarks

In Europe there are many health promotion initiatives, both at a pan-European level and at a national level, that promote a physically active life style, the enhancement of levels of physical fitness, the prevention of sports injuries and the consumption of better nutrition. However, none of these health promotion initiatives combine efforts related to better nutrition, a more physically active lifestyle, and the enhancement of levels of physical fitness. Given the interrelationships between these variables, it is desirable to combine future efforts.

Note

Information on EUROFIT can be obtained from: Council of Europe, Directorate of Education, Culture and Sport, Sports Division, F–67075 Strasbourg Cedex (France); e-mail: suzanne.little@decs.coe.fr.

Information on the 'Europe on the Move' Network can be obtained from: NOC*NSF, PO Box 302, NL–6800 AH Arnhem (The Netherlands); e-mail: international.affairs@noc-nsf.nl;homepage: http//www.noc-nsf/Europe.

References

1   Bouchard C: Physical activity, fitness and health: Overview of the consensus symposium; in Quinney AH, Gauvin L, Wall TA (eds): Toward Active Living. Champaign, Human Kinetics, 1994.
2   Pate RR, Pratt M, Blair SN, Haskell WL, Macera CA, Bouchard C, Buchner D, Ettinger W, Heath GW, King AC, Kriska A, Leon AS, Marcus BH, Morris J, Paffenbarger RS, Patrick K, Pollock ML, Rippe JR, Sallis J, Wilmore JH: Physical activity and public health: A recommendation from the Centers for Disease Control and Prevention and the American College of Sports Medicine. JAMA 1995;273:402–407.
3   Powell KE, Blair SN: The public health burden of sedentary living habits: Theoretical but realistic estimates. Med Sci Sports Exerc 1994;26:851–856.
4   Blair SN, Booth M, Gyarfas I, Iwane H, Matti B, Matsudo V, Marrow MS, Noakes T, Shephard R: The development of public policy and physical activity initiatives internationally. Sports Med 1996;21:157–163.
5   Council of Europe: Recommendation No.R(95)16 of the Committee of Ministers to the Member States on Young People and Sport. Strasbourg, 1995; CDDS (95)58;8–10.
6   Council of Europe: Recommendation No.R(95)17 of the Committee of Ministers to the Member States on the Significance of Sport for Society. Strasbourg, 1995; CDDS (95)58;8–10.
7   Vuori I, Oja P, Stahl T: Promotion of Health-Enhancing Physical Activity. Development of a European strategy, network and action program. Tampere, UKK Institute, 1996.
8   Pyykko M, Paronen O, Oja P, Vuori I: Finland on the Move. Tampere, UKK Institute, 1995.
9   Annonymus: Nota 'Gezond en wel'. Den Haag, SDU, 1995.
10 RIVM (National Institute on Public Health and Environment – Department of Chronic Disease and Environmental Epidemiology): Annual Report. Bilthoven, 1995.
11 van Mechelen W, Hlobil H, Kemper HCG: How can sports injuries be prevented? Oosterbeek, NISGZ, 1987, publ No 25E.

12   van Vulpen A: Sport Injuries and Their Prevention. Papendal, Council of Europe, NISGZ, 1989.
13   van Galen W, Diederiks J: Sportblessures Breed Uitgemeten. Haarlem, De Vrieseborch, 1990.
14   Smikli S, Backx FJG, Bol E: Sportblessures Nader Uitgediept. Houten, BSL, 1995.
15   Adam C, Klissouras V, Ravazzolo M, Renson R, Tukwarth W, Kemper HCG, van Mechelen W, Hlobil M, Bamen G, Levarlet-Joye H (eds): EUROFIT – European Test of Physical Fitness. Council of Europe. Committee for the Development of Sport. Rome, CONI, 1988.
16   Kemper HCG, van Mechelen W: Physical fitness testing of children: A European perspective. J Pediatr Exerc Sci 1996;8:201–214.
17   Oja P, Tuxworth W (eds): Barabas A, Chamarro M, Ekblom B, Levarlet-Joye H, van Mechelen W, Sikarski W: EUROFIT for Adults. Assessment of Health Related Fitness. Strasbourg, Council of Europe/Tampere, UKK Institute, 1995.
18   Vaandrager HW: Constructing a healthy balance: Action and research to facilitate the process of health promotion; PhD-thesis, Wageningen, 1995.
19   Anonymus: Promoting Healthy Eating: The Role of the European Heart Network. Bruxelles, European Community Office, undated brochure.

Willem van Mechelen, MD, PhD, Institute for Research in Extramural Medicine and Department of Social Medicine, Faculty of Medicine, Vrije Universiteit, van der Boechorstraat 7, NL–1081 BT Amsterdam (The Netherlands) e-mail: W.van_Mechelen.EMGO@MED.VU.NL

Simopoulos AP (ed): Nutrition and Fitness: Evolutionary Aspects, Children's Health,
Programs and Policies. World Rev Nutr Diet. Basel, Karger, 1997, vol 81, pp 148–159

....

National Policies Promoting Better Nutrition, Physical Fitness and Sports for All in Australia

A. Stewart Truswell

Human Nutrition Unit, University of Sydney, NSW, Australia

Australia has a relatively small population (16–17 million) widely scattered across a continent but most of the area of Australia is desert or semi-desert and the bulk of the population is concentrated along the coastal strips especially on the east and southeast coast. Politically, the nation of Australia is divided into seven states: New South Wales, Victoria, Queensland, Western Australia, South Australia, Tasmania and the Northern Territory. Each state has its own government responsible, inter alia, for its own hospitals and some other health services. The federal (commonwealth) government is in Canberra in the independent Australian Capital Territory (ACT), analogous to the 'DC' of Washington, USA. Canberra is in the southeast of Australia, inland between Sydney and Melbourne and nearer the former. The federal health department coordinates national health policy and national medical insurance (Medicare and Medibank). The states are jealous of their own semi-autonomy and major national policy decisions on health cannot be made without the agreement of representatives of the states' health departments. Responsibility for sport is also shared, with a federal minister of sport and ministers of sport in each of the states.

Two sections of the federal department of health are most involved in policy and national advice on public health nutrition. The first is the National Health and Medical Research Council (NH&MRC) which convenes expert opinion on health matters, including public health nutrition. For 50 years there was a representative national expert committee on nutrition as part of the NH&MRC structures. Two years ago this was merged into a joint committee on the Environment, Women's Health and Nutrition and the nutrition community feels it has lost the range of expertise and initiative of the NH&MRC nutrition committee, which corresponded to 'COMA' in the UK.

Secondly, food standards come under the federal department of health budget too, looked after by the ANZFA, the Australian and New Zealand Food Authority, housed in a separate building in Canberra. Australia is unusual in that the departments of primary industry (federal and state) that look after agriculture are not primarily responsible for food standards. Australia and New Zealand have this year agreed to a combined national food authority, a practical example of closer economic cooperation across the Tasman Sea.

Another feature of the Australian scene is CSIRO, the Commonwealth Scientific and Industrial Research Organization, which consists of a number of scattered divisions that carry out research in the national interest, on astronomy, meteorology, agriculture, oceanography , fisheries, mining, physics, etc. The CSIRO Division of Human Nutrition in Adelaide (South Australia) has the largest group of nutrition researchers in Australia and acted as host organization for the XV International Nutrition Congress in 1993.

There are also small departments dedicated to human nutrition in some seven of the universities: my own Human Nutrition Unit at the University of Sydney (New South Wales); Deakin University in Geelong and Melbourne (Prof. Kerin O'Dea); Monash University Department of Medicine (Prof. Mark Wahlqvist) also in Melbourne; Curtin University in Perth, West Australia; the University of Queensland (which concentrates on nutritional problems of developing countires), and two new groups at Newcastle University and Wollongong University, both in the state of New South Wales.

Other agencies that play important roles in national advice on nutrition and exercise are the National Heart Foundation of Australia, the Cancer Councils of the different states and two nutrition foundations: the Australian Nutrition Foundation (dedicated to nutrition education of the public) and Sydney University's Nutrition Research Foundation.

The food habits and nutritional problems of Australians are principally those of affluent communities, as in western Europe or north America.

Food and Nutrient Intakes

Apparent consumption figures for foods and the major nutrients are compiled and published each year by the Australian Bureau of Statistics [1].

Individual food intake data were published in the mid-1980s by the Commonwealth Department of Health, for 6,255 adults 25–64 years of age in the state capital cities, based on 24-hour recall [2, 3] and for 5,224 school children aged 10–15 years, based on 24-hour food records [4, 5]. Data was also collected by CSIRO from postal surveys with food frequency questionnaires in Victoria state in 1985 and 1990 [6] and from a national sample of 3,800 in 1988 and 1993 [7]. A National Nutrition Survey with interviews of 13,000 people in their homes has been conducted by the Australian Bureau of Statistics and the Commonwealth Department of Health in 1995. Sampling was based on dwellings across the country: 24-hour recall and food frequency questionnaires were both collected, with simple anthropometry. The subjects ranged from children to old-age pensioners: results should be published in 1997.

Food Composition Analysis

The ANZFA (formerly the national Food Authority) funds what systematic analysis is done on conventional Australian foods and publishes the compiled data. This is available in hard copy as detailed volumes in the *Composition of Foods*, Australia series. It is also available on disk as Nut Tab Australia. A condensed version is published as Nutritional Values of Australian Foods [8]. These conventional foods, except macadamia nuts and the marine fish are not native to the continent. Two university groups and one army laboratory have made a start on analysing Australian 'bush foods', foods that sustained Aboriginal people before Europeans arrived at the end of the eighteenth century. The compilation is published by the Australian Institute of Aboriginal Studies [9].

Groundwork for Present Policies

During the 1980s much of the groundwork was laid for present policies: A subcommittee of the NH&MRC Nutrition Committee produced a major set of Recommended Nutrient Intakes [10] or Recommended Dietary Intakes (RDIs) with explanatory background papers. Unlike many of the RDI reports for small countries, these were (except for protein) not borrowed from FAO/WHO, UK or USA but worked out independently – the process took 7 years. The numbers end up similar to the major international references but there are some interesting details. Sunny Australia has no RDI for vitamin D for the general population; Australia had the first RDI for selenium and was one of the first countries to have RDIs for potassium and sodium.

The RDI for sodium (Na) unlike many RDI numbers, has an upper as well as a lower requirement value. Australians are recommended to eat at least 40 mmol Na but not more than 100 mmol Na/day. This upper recommendation had been reached by another subcommittee of the NH&MRC Nutrition Com-

Table 1. Dietary guidelines for Australians

1981–1991 [17]	1992–present [21]
Promote breast-feeding	Enjoy a wide variety of nutritious foods
Choose a nutritious diet from a variety of foods	Eat plenty of breads and cereal (preferably wholegrain), vegetables (including legumes) and fruits
Control your weight	Eat a diet low in fat and, in particular, low in saturated fat
Avoid eating too much fat	Maintain a healthy body weight by balancing food intake and regular physical activity
Avoid eating too much sugar	If you drink alcohol, limit your intake
Eat more bread and cereals (preferably wholegrain) and vegetables and fruit	Eat only a moderate amount of sugars and foods containing added sugar
Limit alcohol consumption	Choose low salt foods and use salt sparingly
Use less salt	Encourage and support breast-feeding
	Guidelines on specific nutrients Eat foods containing calcium Eat food containing iron

mittee that reported on sodium in the Australian diet [11]. Australia was possibly the first country in the world to publish a recommended upper limit for sodium intake, though it has not yet been achieved by most people [12].

The Australian RDIs are used in New Zealand also, except that the Australian number for selenium (85 µg/day for men and 70 µg/day for women) is too high for New Zealand.

Australia was one of the first countries to adopt the WHO code for breast milk substitutes [13]. Implementation and compliance have been carefully monitored [14]. There has for many years now been public agreement by all sectors that breast-feeding is the basis of infant feeding, and breast-feeding rates are high [15, 16].

The Commonwealth Department of Health produced the first edition of Dietary Guidelines for Australians [17] in 1981. I have elsewhere described the background and reactions to this report, which were nearly all favourable. Australia did not experience the disputes that followed the NACNE report in Britain or 'Dietary Goals' and 'Toward Healthful Diets' in the USA [18]. The headings of the first Australian set of guidelines are shown in table 1.

Governments and all the relevant professional associations – the Australian Dental Association, the Australian Medical Association and scientific nutritionists have all supported fluoridation of water supplies. Sydney's water has been fluoridated since 1968, Canberra's and Hobart's since 1964, Adelaide's since 1971, Melbourne's since 1977.

The Australian National Heart Foundation has been active in encouraging people to eat less saturated fat and replace it with polyunsaturated fat; to limit cholesterol intake, avoid obesity and take regular exercise. The Foundation's Diet and Heart Disease Committee has reviewed the available research data on diet and coronary heart disease at regular intervals from 1971 to 1992 [19]. Australia and the USA have experienced the largest reductions of all countries in age standardized mortality from coronary heart disease (in men and women). The reduction between 1967 and 1993 has been 60% for men in Australia. There has been a corresponding decline in all causes of mortality. At least part of the explanation for this public health success appears to have been the replacement of animal cooking and spreading fats by unsaturated vegetable fats [20].

Australian Nutrition Policy Developments in the 1990s

The NH&MRC dietary guidelines were revised by a representative committee that reported in 1992 [21]. The chairman of the New Zealand Food and Nutrition Taskforce attended the meetings. The second edition of Australian dietary guidelines differs in several ways from the first (table 1). Instead of advising people to avoid eating too much fat, they are now advised to eat a diet low in fat and in particular low in saturated fat. Breast-feeding, though the foundation of healthy nutrition, only applies to one age group so it was moved down the list. Unlike the first edition, the second edition states that the guidelines are in order of priority. Two guidelines were added, emphasizing the importance of calcium and iron for some sections of the community.

Note that these guidelines emphasize what one should eat before what one should cut down. Limitation of fat is now seen as much more important than limitation of sugar. The salt guideline recognizes that most salt intake nowadays come from processed staple foods, rather than the salt shaker. The report of the second edition has a moderate amount of background documentation (much more than in the 20-page first edition).

There have been important products [22] of these evolving Australian dietary guidelines:

(1) Health targets that have been drafted by different committees for the federal Department of Health.

---

(2) Australia's Food and Nutrition Policy [23], a largely political document states in the first paragraph of the policy statement that the goal of the 'policy is to improve health and reduce the preventable burden of diet-related early death, illness and disability among Australians. The policy will be implemented through strategies which support the Australian dietary guidelines, involve key sectors in the food system and foster community participation'...

(3) Posters and food guides. The best known is a pyramid designed by the Australian Nutrition Foundation (for picture see [24]). The concept was later borrowed by the US Department of Agriculture.

(4) Some of the larger food companies now have their own nutrition policies.

(5) Components that feature in the guidelines are included in nutrient labels on foods.

(6) Food products that companies have modified to be closer to the dietary guidelines: reduced fat, reduced saturated fat, reduced salt, reduced calorie, increased fiber foods and reduced alcohol beer.

Because of controversy about different types of fats, the first edition of dietary guidelines avoided specifying type of fat in its heading. But the NH&MRC was asked to provide guidance, so they set up a subcommittee of the nutrition committee to review 'the role of polyunsaturated fats in the Australian diet' [25]. The committee recommended that the target for total fat for individuals should be 30% of energy, with saturated fat 10 en%, polyunsaturated fats 6–10 en%, and replacement of saturated fat with a mix of complex carbohydrates, monounsaturated and polyunsaturated fatty acids. The ratio of n–3 to n–6 polyunsaturated fatty acids should be increased. In infant formulas somewhere around 1:7 (as in human milk) would seem ideal. Trans fatty acids should be considered as saturated fatty acids in relation to their effect on plasma cholesterol.

Confusion continued over different fatty acids and further authoritative reviews were convened by the National Heart Foundation [26] and by the Nutrition Research Foundation (University of Sydney) [27]. The former concentrated on effects on plasma lipids; the latter considered other effects. They largely confirmed recommendations of the NH&MRC Committee and also agreed that n–6 polyunsaturated fatty acids lower plasma cholesterol more than monounsaturated fats.

While the second edition of the dietary guidelines was being drafted, the committee recognized that not all its recommendations apply equally to children. A new committee of pediatricians and some members of the original guidelines committee drafted Dietary Guidelines for Children and Adolescents [28]. The differences from the adult guidelines can be seen in table 2.

Table 2. Australian dietary guidelines

For adults 1992 [21]	For children and adolescents [28]
Enjoy a wide variety of nutritious foods	Encourage and support breast-feeding
Eat plenty of breads and cereals (preferably wholegrain), vegetables (including legumes) and fruits	Children need appropriate food and physical activity to grow and develop normally; growth should be checked regularly
Eat a diet low in fat and, in particular, low in saturated fat	Enjoy a wide variety of nutritious foods
Maintain a healthy body weight by balancing food intake and regular physical activity	Eat plenty of breads and cereals, vegetables (including legumes) and fruits
If you drink alcohol, limit your intake	Low-fat diets are not suitable for young children; for older children, a diet low in fat and, in particular, low in saturated fat is appropriate
Eat only a moderate amount of sugars and foods containing added sugars	Encourage water as a drink; alcohol is not recommended for children
Choose low salt foods and use salt sparingly	Eat only a moderate amount of sugars and foods containing added sugars
Encourage and support breast-feeding	Choose low salt foods
Eat foods containing calcium	Eat foods containing calcium
Eat foods containing iron	Eat foods containing iron

Wernicke-Korsakoff syndrome has been shown to be relatively common in Australia. After several years of discussion (including a proposal to add thiamin to alcoholic beverages) the NH&MRC resolved that it should be mandatory to add thiamin to bread flour as from January 1991. Unlike many other industrial countries Australia had not enriched bread with nutrients up to then. A retrospective survey of in-patient records for all major hospitals in Sydney showed some reduction of Wernicke-Korsakoff admissions in 1992 and 1993 [29].

After publication of the British MRC secondary prevention trial of neural tube defects and the Hungarian primary prevention trial the NH&MRC convened an expert panel to advise on public health policy [30]. Increased folate intake at the time of conception and for 4 weeks after appears to be protective. Nutrition education and folic acid supplements could not reach most women and their embryos. The NH&MRC recommended voluntary fortification with folic acid of stable foods that already carry some folate: all cereal foods, fruit and vegetable juices and yeast extract ('Vegemite'). The National Food Authority changed the food regulations to permit this fortification (at 100 µg folic acid per standard serving). Several breakfast cereals are or soon will be fortified with folic acid. Some men, those with increased plasma homocysteine, may also benefit from this fortification [31].

The latest focus in pubic health nutrition in Australia is on overweight and obesity, which appear to be increasing here, as in other industrial countries, at the same time as coronary heart disease, strokes and all causes of mortality have been declining substantially. The best data is in relatively small samples of adults in state capital cities examined in 1980, 1983 and 1989 by the National Heart Foundation. At the last examination 48% of men and 34% of women aged 25–69 years had body mass indices above 25 [32]. Schoolboys' weights may be increasing too [33]. A committee set up by the NH&MRC is considering and consulting what can be done [34].

Sport and Fitness Policies in Australia

Most Australians are very interested in sport. The next Olympic Games will be in Sydney in AD 2000. Another Australian city, Melbourne, has already hosted the Olympic Games (in 1956). In the recent Atlanta games Australia scored more medals per head of population than any country except Cuba. On 8th August this year 45 thousand people took part in the run from the center of Sydney to Bondi (City to Surf - 14km!) Many suburbs in Australia have their own 'oval', grass field for sport. The mostly sunny, relatively dry climate makes it easy to get outside for exercise. Tennis courts, swimming pools and golf courses are plentiful and for many Australians the sea is near. Federal and state governments have set up institutes of sport, the major one is in Canberra, the Australian Institute of Sport. Australian teams are among the world leaders in cricket and rugby, hockey and basketball (but not yet soccer).

And yet there are reports, documented in the NH&MRC's consultative report [34], that around 30% of the adult population are quite sedentary and do not participate in physical activity. The challenge is to find out more about this group in society and to work out if there are ways in which they can be helped to be more active. There are pressures in complex modern cities which can make it difficult to get regular exercise: illness obviously, not enough time, fear about safety, it's easier and quicker to take the car, the lift, mechanisation in the work place.

Table 3. Food and nutrition guidelines for New Zealand (1991) [35] (for younger adults)

1 Eat a variety of foods from each of the 4 major food groups each day
   Vegetables and fruits
   Breads and cereal foods
   Milks and dairy products, especially the low-fat varieties
   Lean meats, poultry, fish, eggs, nuts or pulses

2 Prepare meals with minimal added fat (especially saturated fat) and salt

3 Choose pre-prepared foods, drinks and snacks that are low in fat (especially saturated fat), salt and sugar

4 Maintain a healthy body weight by regular physical activity and by healthy eating

5 Drink plenty of liquids each day

6 If drinking alcohol do so in moderation

Nutrition Policies in New Zealand

New Zealand is geologically more recent than Australia. It has higher mountains and more fertile soil in its lowlands though the soil is deficient in selenium and iodide. The largest center of population, Auckland, is towards the top end of North Island. The capital, Wellington is at the southern end of North Island. Nutritional expertise is concentrated in Dunedin, far down in South Island, at the University of Otago, which was the first university in the country, set up at the time of the Otago gold rush. The chair of human nutrition at Otago is the oldest in Australasia. The first professor was Marion Robinson, a selenium expert, now retired. The present incumbent is Jim Mann, expert on diabetes and plasma lipids.

The Maoris, a Polynesian people, form a larger proportion of the population than the Aborigines in Australia. Nutrition research has been strong on trace elements and on the nutrition of Pacific Islanders.

The first of a recent series of reports on food and nutrition policy for New Zealand, the report of the Nutrition Taskforce [35] (chaired by Prof. Cliff Tasman-Jones), appeared in 1991. In 189 pages it considered all aspects of the food system and nutrition education, legislation, food quality and safety, surveillance and research, economic implications). It proposes a set of dietary guidelines (table 3) and in the last chapter sets out a list of 423 strategies.

While the Australian federal department of health has produced a new dietary guidelines report for adults and another for children and adolescents in the 1990s, the New Zealand Public Health Commission has produced five different age-specific reports [36–40].

Each of these is a substantial publication of 40 to 50 pages. The guidelines are different for each subgroup. For example, for the older people the headings are: eat a variety of foods; keep active and maintain a healthy weight; choose foods low in fat, sugar and salt; have plenty to drink; go easy on alcohol; make mealtime a social time – where possible.

The New Zealand health authorities and their nutritional consultants are thus following a policy recommended at a WHO meeting in Japan [41], that we should try to move to a single set of dietary reference values for essential nutrients – New Zealand has adopted the Australian RDIs except for selenium and iodine [35]. But for amounts and types of fat, carbohydrates and other non-essential dietary components, dietary guidelines will be most effective if the target group is defined.

Another important document is the 'National Plan of Action for Nutrition' [42], prepared in response to the International Conference on Nutrition (ICN) Rome 1992. It was published in 1995 and is unusually clear and well set out for a report of this type. The plans are presented under three of the headings of the ICN: improving household food security; improving food quality and safety, and promoting appropriate diets and healthy lifestyles.

Last, a National Nutrition Survey is being actively planned at present. It will be funded by the government, directed by Prof. David Russell of LINZ (Life in New Zealand), University of Otago. The survey will include samples of Maori people and Pacific Islanders living in New Zealand. In contrast to the recent Australian survey, this survey will include blood and urine analyses.

References

1   Madden R: Apparent Consumption of Foodstuffs and Nutrients, Australia 1992–93. Canberra, Australian Bureau of Statistics, 1995.
2   Commonwealth Department of Health: National Dietary Survey of Adults: 1983. No 1. Foods Consumed. Canberra, Australian Government Publishing Service, 1986.
3   Department of Community Services of Health: National Dietary Survey of Adults:1983.No.2. Nutrient intakes. Canberra, Australian Government Publishing Service, 1987.
4   Department of Community Services and Health: National Dietary Survey of Schoolchildren (aged 10–15 years): 1985. No 1. Foods Consumed. Canberra, Australian Government Publishing Service, 1988.
5   Department of Community Services and Health: National Dietary Survey of Schoolchildren (aged 10–15 years): 1985. No 2. Nutrient Intakes. Canberra, Australian Government Publishing Service, 1989.
6   CSIRO Division of Human Nutrition: What Are Australians eating? Results from the 1985 and 1990 Victorian Nutrition Surveys. Adelaide, CSIRO Division of Human Nutrition, 1993.

7   CSIRO Division of Human Nutrition: Food and Nutrition in Australia – does Five Years Make a Difference? Results from the CSIRO Australian Food and Nutrition Surveys 1988 and 1993. Adelaide, CSIRO Australian Division of Human Nutrition, 1996.
8   English R, Lewis J: Nutritional Values of Australian Foods. Canberra, Australian Government Publishing Service, 1991.
9   Brand Miller JC, James K, Maggiore P: Tables of Composition of Australian Aboriginal Foods. Canberra, Australian Institute of Aboriginal and Torres Straight Islanders, 1993.
10 Truswell AS, Dreosti IE, English RM,Rutishauser IHE, Palmer N: Recommended Nutrient Intakes, Australian Papers. Mosman, Sydney, Australian Professional Publications, 1990.
11 Morgan TO, Hosking M, Scoggins BA, Truswell AS, Cornish M, West C: Report of the NH&MRC Working Party on Sodium in the Australian Diet. Canberra, Australian Government Publishing Service, 1994.
12 Notowidjojo L, Truswell AS: Urinary sodium and potassium in a sample of healthy adults in Sydney, Australia. Asia Pacific J Clin Nutr 1993;25–33.
13 National Health and Medical Research Council: Report of the Working Party on Implementation of the WHO International Code on Marketing of Breast Milk Substitutes. Canberra, Australian Government Publishing, 1985.
14 Commonwealth Department of Health, Housing and Community Services: Review of the Implementation in Australia of the WHO International Code of Marketing of Breast Milk Substitutes. Canberra, Commonwealth Department of Health, Housing and Community Services, 1993.
15 Palmer N: Breast feeding – the Australian situation. J Food Nutr (Canberra) 1985;42:13–18.
16 Lester IH: Australia's Food and Nutrition. Australian Institute of Health and Welfare. Canberra, Australian Government Publishing Service, 1994.
17 Commonwealth Department of Community Services and Health: Dietary Guidelines for Australians. Canberra, Australian Government Publishing Service, 1981.
18 Truswell AS: Objectives and uses of dietary guidelines with emphasis on the Australian experience; in Latham MC, van Veen MS (eds): Dietary Guidelines: Proceedings of an International Conference, Toronto, 1988. Cornell University Int Nutr Monogr Ser No 21, 1989.
19 Shrapnel WS, Calvert GD, Nestel PJ, Truswell AS: Diet and coronary heart disease: A position statement of the National Heart Foundation of Australia. Med J Aust 1992; 152 (suppl May 4).
20 Lloyd B: Declining cardiovascular disease incidence and environmental components. Aust NZ J Med 1994;24:124–132.
21 National Health and Medical Research Council: Dietary Guidelines for Australians, ed 2. Canberra, Australian Government Publishing Service, 1992.
22 Truswell AS: Dietary guidelines: Theory and practice. Proc Nutr Soc Aust 1995;19:1–10.
23 Commonwealth Department of Health, Housing and Community Services: Food and Nutrition Policy. Canberra, Australian Government Publishing Service, 1992.
24 Truswell AS: Evolution of dietary recommendations, goals and guidelines. Am J Clin Nutr 1987; 45:1060–1070.
25 Truswell AS, Craske JD, English R, Nestel PJ, Sinclair A, Lester IH, Lilburne AM: The Role of Polyunsaturated Fats in the Australian Diet. Report of the NH&MRC Working Party. Canberra, Australian Government Publishing Service, 1992.
26 Shrapnel WS, Truswell AS, Nestel PJ, Simons LA: Dietary Fatty Acids and Blood Cholesterol. Canberra, National Heart Foundation of Australia, 1994.
27 Truswell AS, Laws OWR, Kefford JF (eds): Which Fatty Acids? University of Sydney Nutrition Research Foundation Annual Symposium. Food Australia 1995; (March suppl):S1–S31.
28 Binns C, Carmichael A, Cashel K, Coles-Rutishauser I, Davidson G, Spencer S, Truswell AS, Warden R, van Belkon P, Jefferson S: Dietary Guidelines for Children and Adolescents. Canberra, National Health & Medical Research Council, 1995.
29 Ma JJ, Truswell AS: Wernicke-Korsakoff syndrome in Sydney hospitals: Before and after thiamine enrichment of flour. Med J Aust 1995;163:531–534.
30 Report of the Expert Panel: Folate Fortification. Canberra, National Health & Medical Research Council, 1995.

31   Truswell AS (ed):Folate, malformations, homocysteinaemia and folic acid in our foods. Aust J Nutr Diet 1996;53(June suppl):S1–S35.
32   National Heart Foundation of Australia: Risk Factor Prevalence Study. Survey No 3, 1989. Canberra, National Heart Foundation and Australian Institute of Health, 1990.
33   Wilcken DEL, Lynch JF, Marshall MD, et al: Relevance of body weight to apolipoprotein levels in Australian childrent. Med J Aust 1996;164:22–25.
34   Acting on Australia's Weight: A Strategy for the Prevention of Overweight and Obesity. Draft for Public Comment. Canberra, National Health & Medical Research Council, 1996.
35   The Report of the Nutrition Taskforce: Food for Health. Wellington, Department of Health (Te Tari Ora), 1991.
36   Reid J, George J, Pears R: Food and Nutrition Guidelines for Children Aged 2–12 Years. Wellington, Department of Health (Te Tari Ora), 1992.
37   Food and Nutrition Guidelines for New Zealand Adolescents: A Background Paper. Wellington, Public Health Commission (Rangapu Hanora Tumatanui),1993.
38   Food and Nutrition Guidelines for Infants and Toddlers (from birth to two years of age). Wellington, Department of Health, 1994.
39   Food and Nutrition Guidelines for Healthy Pregnant Women: A Background Paper (major author Joanne Todd). Wellington, Public Health Commission (Rangapu Hanora Tumatanui), 1995.
40   Food and Nutrition Guidelines for Healthy Older People: A Background Paper (written by Caroline Horwath). Wellington, Ministry of Health (Manatu Hanora), 1996.
41   Pietinen P, Truswell AS: Highlights from the Second WHO Symposium on Health Issues for the 21st Century: Nutrition and Quality of Life (Kobe, Japan, November 1993). Geneva, World Health Organization Programme, 1994.
42   National Plan of Action for Nutrition: The Public Health Commission's Advise to the Minister of Health 1994–1995. Wellington, Public Health Commission (Rangapu Hanora Tumatanni), 1995.

A. Stewart Truswell, Human Nutrition Unit, The University of Sydney,
Sydney, NSW 2006 (Australia)

Simopoulos AP (ed): Nutrition and Fitness: Evolutionary Aspects, Children's Health,
Programs and Policies. World Rev Nutr Diet. Basel, Karger, 1997, vol 81, pp 160–166

Is Physical Activity Promotion on the Primary Health Care Agenda?

Mairi M. Gould[a], Steve Iliffe[a], Margaret Thorogood[b]

[a] Department of Primary Care and Population Sciences, University College London
Medical School and Royal Free Hospital School of Medicine, and
[b] Health Promotion Sciences Unit, London School of Hygiene and Tropical Medicine,
London, UK

In the UK a key priority of the 'Health of the Nation' [1] document is prevention of coronary heart disease (CHD). Recent findings suggest that low physical activity levels contribute to CHD risk [2] and the 1992 Allied Dunbar National Fitness Survey confirmed that physical activity levels are low in England [3] with around 70% of adults taking insufficient exercise to confer a health benefit.

There have been many changes in the health care system in recent years with a shift in emphasis in primary care from a curative to a health promotion model. However, little training or support has been given to primary health care teams (PHCTs) in promoting physical activity [4, 5]. The Health Education Authority (HEA) has developed a guide [6] to enable PHCTs to develop a systematic approach to assessment and promotion of physical activity. An evaluation of this guide was carried out during November and December 1994, prior to the final version being drafted.

Background to the guide: The draft guide contained detailed information about the health benefits of exercise, including an update on the most recent research findings.

It also included a 'framework for agreeing a practice policy' which suggested: calling a practice meeting brainstorming ideas around health promotion and how physical activity could be incorporated into current practice; setting tasks; and developing a practice policy.

The Prochaska and DiClemente [7] model of change was outlined as a means of assessing the individual patient's readiness to adopt a behaviour change. There was a section on the legal aspects of promotion of physical activity which stated that GPs have clinical responsibility for any patient to whom they recommended increasing their activity levels.

Three levels of exercise promotion were described:

Level 1: Opportunistic advice about the health benefits of exercise.

Level 2: Counselling about exercise and fitness, by trained staff, in dedicated time.

Level 3: An exercise programme, established in house or by arrangement with local sports and leisure facilities.

Sample Frame

In order to evaluate the guide, we chose a sample frame with the following sources:

(1) Training practices in the North and South Thames Regions. Trainers are likely to be aware of developments in primary health care and issues around changing behaviour, as part of the preparation required for accreditation.

(2) Teaching practices in the UCLMS/Royal Free network. Most of these include lectures in primary care, and range from inner-city to outer suburban in character.

(3) Practices which participated in the OXCHECK study. Staff in these had previous experience of testing a health promotion programme.

Practices were approached initially by a letter to the GP, followed within a few days by a telephone call, to obtain a sample of practices that can be categorised as: (a) inner-city/suburban/rural; (b) single handed/small (2–4 GPs)/ large (5 or more GPs), and (c) fundholder/non-fundholder.

The practices chosen were confined to the southeast of England because of time and financial constraints. Those practices agreeing to participate were sent three copies of the guide, to be reviewed by one (or more) doctors, one (or more) practice nurses and the practice manager (or other reception staff, if appropriate). Reviewers were asked to annotate the guides anonymously.

The Research Method

The practices were visited by the fieldworker (M.G.), who conducted semi-structured one-to-one interviews with different categories of staff, except in one practice, where the general practitioner and nurse were interviewed together. Interviews were tape recorded, and transcribed verbatim. Transcriptions were analysed systematically by two researchers (M.G. and S.I.).

Table 1. Characteristics of the 11 participating practices

Number of GP partners		Situation of practice	
Single-handed	1	Inner-city	4
2–4 partners	6	Suburban	6
5 or more partners	4	Rural	1
Fundholding status		Level of funding	
Fundholding	3	Band three funding	10
Non-fundholding	8	Lower level funding	1

This evaluation study used three qualitative research techniques: stratified purposeful sampling; semi-structured interviewing; and systematic text analysis.

Interview Content

The interview was based around the main sections of the guide, using open questions, followed by specific prompts. The following topics were covered:

(1) The strength of the argument for promoting exercise in primary care.

(2) The applicability of the definitions of moderate and vigorous activity in the primary care setting.

(3) The feasibility of encouraging exercise through primary care, including potential costs and opportunity costs.

(4) The implications for staff training, practice organisation and finances of exercise promotion programmes.

(5) The risks and legal liabilities associated with exercise promotion, including the applicability of a risk stratification protocol.

(6) The perceived relevance of the Prochaska and DiClemente model to exercise behaviour in the local population.

Results

Thirty-eight practices were approached and 18 agreed to participate. Twelve of these were chosen to fit the desired sample, but one was subsequently unable to take part within the project timescale.

The characteristics of the 11 participating practices are shown in table 1. One of the three fundholding practices had already developed an exercise

Table 2. Comments about difficulties in assessing activity levels

---

'People under- or overestimate what they do'
'People aren't honest'
'I think they mislead you'
'They all fib about what they do'
'I don't know how reliable their answers are'
'People have false notions'
'They tell us what they plan to do, not what they are doing'

---

promotion scheme with dedicated staff. In this practice, the exercise instructor was interviewed instead of a practice nurse and in another (non-fundholding) practice, the practice osteopath was interviewed instead of a doctor. Ten GPs, ten nurses, seven managers, one exercise instructor and one osteopath were interviewed.

Promoting Physical Activity Through Primary Care

There was agreement that physical activity is good for health but mixed views on the appropriateness of primary health care as a venue for its promotion. One GP commented, 'If we don't do it, who is going to do it?' and the osteopath thought that it was 'probably the most obvious place'. However, there was dissent (from two GPs, three nurses and one manager). One GP said, 'I'd have to be much more convinced about the health benefits'. The others raised concerns at ideological and practical levels – about 'medicalising a lifestyle change' and about the shortage of resources. One GP commented that PHC is one of several venues, not the only one for promoting physical activity. Eight of the participants talked about physical activity in health promotion terms and sixteen saw it as therapy for specific complaints. One nurse noted that from recent medical and nursing journals, 'there is a clear indication that exercise *does* promote health'. One GP said, 'I've been advocating exercise to patients since I've been a doctor. The body was designed for exercise and if we don't use the body for what it was intended, it's going to complain and object.' Another GP was concerned that the distinction between individual patient care and public health measures was not clear in the guide.

Assessing Current Activity Levels

All the interviewees found it difficult to assess patients' activity levels; a range of the comments made are shown in table 2. All except two of the GPs found the framework for assessing patients' current activity levels helpful.

Costs

All participants anticipated extra costs if an organised scheme for promoting physical activity were to be implemented in their practice. Almost all raised concerns about lack of staff, time and space. Reimbursement was raised as a problem by GPs and managers, who were not convinced that dedicated staff could be paid for in the current situation in general practice. One GP was reluctant to put more resources in until there was more evidence about the efficacy of physical activity promotion in the primary care setting. Another manager commented, 'I'm afraid that the government's idea is that they want us to do the work, but they're not willing to provide the funds… . I think it would need to be a project that was funded… and maybe it could be piloted by a few practices – with some proper research to see what the results really were.'

Setting Up a Physical Activity Promotion Programme

At least one member of every practice felt that promotion of physical activity was already being undertaken, either at registration and other (usually nurse-led) 'health checks', or opportunistically, during consultations. This can be regarded as the equivalent of 'level 1' in the guide. One practice manager commented that level 3 was a good idea because 'it transfers responsibility to the patient'. Comments from two of the GPs suggested that they thought level 3 was a good idea but unlikely to happen because of the amount of long term planning and extra resources needed. One GP was 'not convinced about health promotion in general'.

Opinions were divided over the 'framework for agreeing a practice policy'; five GPs, seven nurses and one manager thought it overambitious and impractical because it would involve practice meetings and potentially lengthy discussions.

Amongst those who were not averse to a change in policy, lack of resources was seen as a barrier. Those who were interested in implementing an exercise programme (five GPs, three nurses, two managers) regarded this as a task for the future.

Five GPs, eight nurses, the osteopath and one manager said they would opt for a level one programme. Only three GPs and one manager said they would consider level three and they all indicated that this would not be possible for several years and, even then, only if resources were available.

Prochaska and DiClemente's Model of Behaviour Change

Seven GPs, six nurses, one manager and the exercise instructor said they were familiar with or had some awareness of the Prochaska and DiClemente model. Eight GPs, seven nurses and four managers thought it was a useful model for understanding behaviour.

The main criticism of this model of behaviour change was that it would be too time consuming for routine use in consultations. One GP pointed out that it was essentially descriptive and did not act as a guide to changing behaviour. The same GP also commented that the model had been described as a linear progression, comparable to a curative process, rather than as a cyclic process containing possibilities of relapse and subsequent renewed enthusiasm. (This was primarily due to the way it was set out in the draft guide.)

Legal Aspects of Exercise Promotion

All participants found a review of the legal liabilities around exercise promotion useful, but only two GPs accepted the issues outlined without anxiety. One of the GPs thought that the lengthy emphasis on legal liabilities was indicative of the over-intrusion of general practice into people's lives. Comments from the others ranged from 'a minor problem' to 'terrifying' because the responsibility for patient safety lies with the GP if she/he has prescribed a course of physical activity.

One nurse expressed concern that nurses also may be legally liable; the exercise instructor already had her own indemnity insurance. All the managers were worried by the legal issues, with one commenting that legal complexities would make an exercise scheme 'not feasible' in her practice.

Discussion

We deliberately chose an atypical group of practices with teaching, training, research or advanced health promotion features in order to test this guide in an environment receptive to new ideas and the possibility of change. While the response from this group is not necessarily generalisable, a positive response should indicate that there is an important group of primary care staff who are ready to take promotion of physical activity seriously. A negative response from this group would suggest that the message of this guide is not likely to be taken up by other primary care staff.

In this selected group we found a readiness to contemplate the adoption of physical activity promotion schemes and previous work has indicated that practice nurses are particularly enthusiastic about this [8]. The group was unhappy about issues of legal liability and about the resource implications of any approach other than opportunistic health promotion. Their enthusiasm for, and lack of knowledge about, assessing current activity, understanding behaviour change, and risk assessment suggest that the opportunistic promotion of physical activity currently undertaken is quite superficial. If this group of practices represent those ready for change, education about opportunistic health promotion is still the greatest need. Particular emphasis should be placed on assessing current activity levels, and on applying models of behaviour change in consultations.

Conclusion

Promotion of physical activity is only just on the Primary Health Care agenda. Concerns over medicalisation of lifestyle are not new [9], and the public health issue of responsibility for primary prevention and the suitability of primary care for this is unresolved. Resources will be needed both to enhance the understanding that primary care staff have about the health benefits of exercise, and to enable them to apply that understanding in practice. Fundholding practices may be able to find resources to employ new staff and obtain dedicated space for ambitious activity programmes but, even opportunistic promotion of physical activity will need more education resources than are currently available to PHCTs.

Acknowledgement

This evaluation was funded by the Health Education Authority. We would also like to thank all the participating practices for their time and input to the project.

References

1   The Health of the Nation: London, Department of Health, 1990.
2   Berlin JA, Colditz GA: A meta-analysis of physical activity in the prevention of coronary heart disease. Am J Epidemiol 1990;132:612–628.
3   Allied Dunbar National Fitness Survey: A Report on Activity Patterns and Fitness Levels. Commissioned by the Sports Council and Health Education Authority. London, 1992.
4   Gould MM, Thorogood M, Morris JN, Iliffe S: Promoting exercise in primary care. Br J Gen Pract 1995;45:159–160.
5   Gould MM, Thorogood M, Iliffe S, Morris JN: Promoting physical activity in primary care: Measuring the knowledge gap. Health Educ J 1995;54:304–311.
6   Promoting Physical Activity through Primary Care: A Guide to Setting Up a Programme. London, HEA, 1996.
7   Prochaska JO, DiClemente CC: Towards a comprehensive model of change; in Miller WR, Heather N (eds): Treating Addictive Behaviors: Processes of Change, New York, Plenum, 1986.
8   Gould MM, Iliffe S, Thorogood M, Morris JN: Promoting physical activity in primary care: Differences between general practitioners and practice nurses. Submitted.
9   Williams SJ, Calnan M: Perspectives on prevention: The views of general practitioners. Sociol Health Illness 1994;16:372–393.

Mairi Gould, Faculty of Health Care Sciences, St. George's Hospital Medical School and Kingston University, Grosvenor Wing, St. George's Hospital, Blackshaw Road, Tooting, London SW17 0QT (UK)

Author Index

Bouchard, C. 72
Bourne, P.G. 105

Chen, J.D. 114
Cordain, L. 26, 49

Eaton, S.B. 24, 26, 49

Gagnon, J. 72
Gotshall, R.W. 49
Gould, M.M. 160
Grave, G.D. 84

Iliffe, S. 160

Lee, P.R. 13, 108
Leon, A.S. 72

Matalas, A.-L. 128
Meyers, L.D. 13, 108

Oja, P. 98

Phillipson, C. 38

Rao, D.C. 72

Siandwazi, C. 122
Simopoulos, A.P. 24, 61
Skinner, J.S. 72
Stallings, V.A. 90

Thorogood, M. 160
Truswell, A.S. 148

van Mechelen, W. 136

Wilmore, J.H. 72

Subject Index

Africa
  micronutrient deficiencies 123, 124
  nutrition and fitness programs
    achievements 125, 126
    development and implementation 124,
      125
    government role 122, 123
    monitoring 126
    overview 106
  protein energy malnutrition 123, 124
Alcohol
  associated health problems 31
  energy in diet 31
Apo E
  genetic variation and dietary response of
    cholesterol levels 66–68
  isoforms 65
  phenotypes 66
Apo IV, genetic variation and dietary
  response of cholesterol levels 68
Australia
  food
    composition analysis 150
    intake 149, 150
  geography and government 148
  nutrition and fitness programs
    dietary guidelines 151–155
    fatty acid classification 153

government agencies and role 148,
  149
nutrition education in universities 149
sports and fitness 155
water fluoridation 152
obesity prevalence 155
Recommended Dietary Intakes 150, 151,
  157
supplementation
  folate 154,155
  thiamin 154

Bone mineral density
  children and exercise 86, 88, 89, 99
  osteoporosis screening 96
  physical activity effects 57, 58
Breast feeding, education in China 117

Carbohydrate, effect on appetite 38
Carrot, development as food 43
Cereal grains, nutritional value 28
Children
  bone mineral density and exercise 86, 88,
    89, 99
  calcium intake in girls 85
  fitness parameters 87, 89, 100, 101
  health benefits of exercise 85, 86, 90, 98,
    99, 102

nutritional needs of exercising child
  energy needs 91
  fluid needs 96
  minerals 96
  overview 84, 85
  Recommended Dietary Allowance 91
  resting energy expenditure
    prediction 85, 91–95
obesity
  exercise prevention 99
  racial differences 88
  trends 89, 102
physical education recommendations 87,
  88, 101
self-reported activity assessment 86, 87,
  100, 101
China
  agricultural production 114
  food consumption 114, 118
  growth retardation of children 115, 116
  nutrition and fitness programs
    breast feeding education 117
    Chinese Nutrition Society
      recommendations 118, 119
    overview 106
    policy goals 120
    Soybean Action 117
    Sports for All plan 119, 120
  prevalence of chronic diseases 118
  vitamin A supplementation 117
Concept of Positive Health
  diagrammatic visualization 2
  Hippocratic statement 1, 2, 13, 61
Cretan diet
  history 131, 132
  longevity effects 42, 43, 46, 47,
    132
  westernization trend 132, 133

Dairy products
  milk allergy 29
  nutritional value 29
Declaration of Olympia on Nutrition and
  Fitness, *see* International Conference on
  Nutrition and Fitness
Diabetes, insulin sensitivity effects of
  exercise 56, 57

Diet, *see also* specific foods
  barriers to health in industrialized
    countries 19, 20
  chronic disease prevention 14
  education 5, 6
  hunter-gatherer diet
    energy intake 31, 32
    fat 29, 30, 33, 39
    micronutrients 32
    paleonutrition recommendations 35,
      36, 46, 47
    salt 30
    wild game 28, 33, 34
    wild vegetal foods 27, 34
  macronutrients 3, 4
  micronutrients 4
  policy development in United States
    government role 105
    history 15–18
    progress in implementation 18, 19
    recommendations 16, 17
Dietary Guidelines for Americans, history of
  development 16–18

Energy, ancestral vs modern human
  intake 31, 32, 55
EUROFIT, *see* Europe
Europe, nutrition and fitness programs
  EUROFIT initiative
    adults
      aims 142–144
      test battery 143, 144
    children test battery 141
  Europe against Cancer program 145
  Europe on the Move
    implementation 140
    recommendations 138, 139
  European Heart Network 145
  Finland on the Move program 139
  information gathering for policy
    development 137
  integration of programs 146
  joint research projects on nutrition 144,
    145
  overview 107
  physical activity recommendations by
    Committee of Ministers 138

Europe (continued)
sports injury prevention programs 140,
141
The Netherlands
nutrition programs 144
physical fitness programs 140
United Kingdom, *see* United Kingdom
Exercise, *see* Physical activity

Fat
ancestral vs modern human intake 29, 30,
33, 39
effect on appetite 38, 39
energy content 39
polyunsaturated fatty acid effects on gene
expression 63
Fiber, ancestral vs modern human intake
27, 34
Finland, *see* Europe
Flour, nutritional value 30
Folate, supplementation in Australia 154,
155

Genetic variation
dietary response 65–69
evolution in man 26
human populations and behavioral effects
2, 3
molecular biology tools 61, 63
polymorphic variation frequency 62
Glycemic index, ancient vs modern foods
43, 44, 47
Greece, *see also* Cretan diet
dietary trends 131–133
nutrition and fitness programs
government role 133, 134
history 128, 129
nutrition education 133, 134
overview 106
physical education in schools 129,
130
Sports for All program 130
success of programs 131
sports heritage 128

Heart rate, fitness parameter in children
87, 89, 100, 101

HERITAGE Family Study, genetic variation
of exercise response
aims 74
cell line maintenance 77, 78
data analysis
association studies 80
linkage analysis 80
path analysis 79
segregation analysis 79, 80
data entry 78
design 75
measurements
anthropometric measurements 76
blood pressure 76
exercise tests 76
glucose tolerance test 77
lipids and lipoproteins 77
serum steroids 77
sampling 75
training program 78

International Conference on Nutrition and
Fitness
conference resolutions of 1988 meeting 12
Declaration of Olympia on Nutrition and
Fitness
distribution 7, 8
1992 meeting 10, 11
1996 meeting 6, 7
proceedings 1
strategies for better health activism 20, 21

Kidney, diet and disease 40, 41

Life span
ancient vs modern man 41–43
Cretan diet effects 42, 43, 132
Lipoprotein lipase, exercise effects on
gene expression 63, 64
Low-density lipoprotein
exercise effects on size 69
subclass patterns and dietary response 68

Meat
fatty acid types 29
nutritional value of game animals vs
commercial meat 28, 29, 33, 34

New Zealand
  geography 156
  nutritional policies 156, 157
Nitric oxide synthase, exercise effects on
  gene expression 65

Obesity
  Australia prevalence 155
  children
    exercise prevention 99
    racial differences 88
    trends 89, 102
  sedentary lifestyle association 136
Osteoporosis, *see* Bone mineral density

Paleonutrition, modern recommendations
  35, 36, 46, 47
Parsnip, development as food 43, 44
Physical activity
  barriers to health in industrialized
    countries 19, 20
  bone mineral density effects 57, 58
  children, *see* Children
  chronic disease prevention 14, 15
  education, *see* Physical education
  effects on gene expression
    lipoprotein lipase 63, 64
    nitric oxide synthase 65
  energy requirements, evolution 31, 32, 55,
    56
  genetic variation in response
    factors affecting response 73
    study, *see* HERITAGE Family Study
  hominid anatomy/physiology, changes
    impacting exercise capabilities
    bipedalism and energy expenditure
      50–52
    body enlargement 53–55
    cranial capacity 52, 53
    hominid-pongid divergence 49, 50
    main events of evolution 50
    thermoregulation 52
  insulin sensitivity effects 56, 57
  low-density lipoprotein size
    dependence 69
  maximal oxygen uptake adaptation 73
  overall health impact 4, 5, 72, 137, 138

policy development by government 19
  types 5
Physical education, *see also* specific
  countries and programs
  media campaigns 5, 6
  recommendations for children 87, 88,
    101
Positive health, *see* Concept of Positive
  Health
Processed food, nutritional value 30, 31
Prochaska and DiClemente's model of
  behavior change, health worker awareness
  164, 165
Protein
  ancestral vs modern human intake 33, 34,
    40, 41
  nutritional value of game animals vs
    commercial meat 28, 29, 33

Resting energy expenditure
  indirect calorimetry measurement 93, 94
  prediction of nutritional needs of
    exercising child 85, 91–95

Salt, ancestral human diet 30, 32
Smoking, trends in industrialized countries
  19, 20
Soybean Action, goals and implementation
  in China 117
Sports for All program
  China 119, 120
  Greece 130
Sports injury, prevention programs in
  Europe 140, 141
Steatopygia, evolution 39

The Netherlands, *see* Europe
Thiamin, supplementation in Australia 154
Tobacco, *see* Smoking
Tryptophan, dietary components and levels
  in brain 40

United Kingdom
  primary health care team promotion of
    physical activity, evaluation of guide
    activity level assessment 163, 166
    background of contents 160, 161

United Kingdom (continued)
  compliance of health care workers in
    promotion 163, 165
  cost concerns 164, 166
  interview content 162
  legal liability concerns 165
  Prochaska and DiClemente's model of
    behavior change 164, 165
  program development attitudes 164
  research method 161, 162
  sample frame 161
  Strategy Statement on Physical Activity
    139, 140
United States, nutrition and fitness programs
  food safety 112
  food service and healthy food choices 111

health professional role in education 111
media campaigns 5, 6, 109
nutrition labeling 111, 112
nutritional policy development
  government role 105,109–113
  history 15–18
  progress in implementation 18, 19
  recommendations 16, 17
private sector partnerships 110
research and surveillance studies 112, 113

Vanadium, manic behavior etiology in
  ancient Greece 44, 45
Vitamin A, supplementation in China 117
Vitamins, ancestral vs modern human
  intake 32